ERRATUM

Page 92, line 16: The following sentence should be inserted
before the sentence beginning "This is a wound. . .":
The attack occurs when the artery completely blocks
so that no blood reaches the area of heart muscle,
resulting in the death of cells (infarct).

HEART ATTACK!

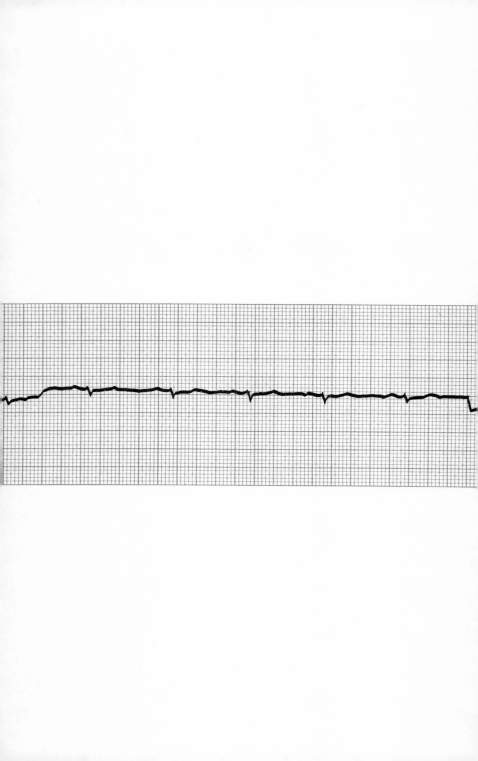

HEART ATTACK!

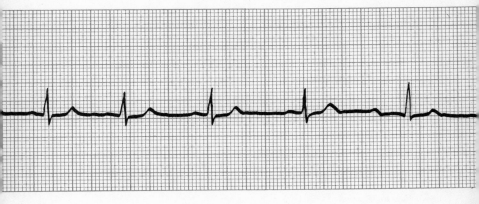

LOUIS S. LEVINE

HARPER & ROW, PUBLISHERS
New York Hagerstown San Francisco London

FIRST EDITION

Designed by Patricia Dunbar

Library of Congress Cataloging in Publication Data

Levine, Louis S
  Heart attack!

    1. Heart—Infarction—Personal narratives.
2. Levine, Louis S. I. Title.
RC685.I6L44 1976   616.1′23′09 [B]   75–30337
ISBN 0–06–012595–0

---

76 77 78 79 10 9 8 7 6 5 4 3 2 1

To my wife, Hannah,
and my children

CONTENTS

ACKNOWLEDGMENTS

An author never writes a book by himself. People, places, facts and circumstances all share in writing the story. Like every other author, I am grateful to those persons who have assisted me—those but for whom this book could never have been written:

My wife, Hannah, who endured so much that I should live.

Steven, Robert, Danette and Suzanne, my four children, who, together with my wife, were responsible for my choosing life instead of death—a choice I have never regretted.

A true friend, Philip Lanzkowsky, M.D., who gave so unselfishly of his time and was always available when I most needed him.

Howard Adelman, M.D., another unselfish friend, who followed my case and gave my wife hope during her moments of despair. Once when I was depressed and in great pain, he appeared miraculously at my bedside to encourage me.

My family, neighbors and friends, too numerous to mention by name.

To all of these wonderful people who contributed to the writing of this chronicle, I express my heartfelt gratitude.

"Yea, though I walk through the valley of the shadow of death, I will fear no evil: for thou art with me . . ."

Psalms 23:4

PREFACE

The writing of this book was conceived while I was a patient in the intensive care unit at a large metropolitan medical center. While recovering from a stroke which had temporarily paralyzed the right side of my body, and affected my speech center and throat muscles so that I could neither speak nor swallow, I suffered a heart attack that was supposed to be fatal. Thank God that no other part of my brain was damaged, and my mind was totally unaffected. Unable to read, talk or move about, I passed the time by thinking about everything that had just happened to me. Surprisingly, I could fathom or comprehend few of the emotional and physiological aspects of either of my afflictions.

During the afterperiod of convalescence, my wife visited the local library and returned home with many books written about heart attacks for lay consumption. The more I read, the angrier I became at my own ignorance and lack of information. I decided then to research and write this book so that other laymen could be better informed than I was, and perhaps, through this knowledge, seek early medical assistance if it seemed advisable.

Thus this book began as a mental exercise as I lay in a hospital bed; the research started when I hungered for knowledge; and the actual writing was launched as a crusade to educate and possibly to save the lives of some of the millions of people who are presently unknowingly afflicted, as I was, with diseased coronary arteries that will eventually produce heart attacks.

1 PUBLIC ENEMY NUMBER ONE

If I had been told that I was a statistical candidate for coronary artery disease and would eventually have a severe heart attack, I wouldn't have believed it.

During the first thirty-nine years of my existence, I always considered myself to be in excellent health. I hadn't been subject to many childhood diseases, although at eight my appendix was removed. Perhaps I was one or two inches shorter than the average at five feet eight and a half inches, stocky, about twenty pounds overweight, sedentary and lethargic (not liking to exert myself physically or exercise regularly), and maybe I couldn't curb my appetite for steaks, chops, spaghetti and sweets. But then I wasn't sickly either.

At thirty-nine years of age, I was entering that plateau most Americans call "the prime of life." I was young enough to reach for the stars, sufficiently aggressive and ambitious to attain my goals, old enough to know better, but too immature to appreciate and enjoy what I possessed.

My wife, my four young children and I lived in a suburb of New York and enjoyed the spaciousness of our split-level house. I loved donning shorts or dungarees, walking barefoot through a thick carpet of green grass, picnicking just outside our kitchen door, or lying beneath a tall tree with bits of blue sky peeping through the leafy branches every now and then.

15

But—not such joys—lawns had to be fertilized and mowed regularly, snow had to be shoveled and removed, painting and repairs always had to be done, the children constantly had to be driven to and from their various community activities, and the mortgage, taxes and bills had to be paid.

Everything considered, I actually had little time to enjoy my home and family. I spent long hours in my New York office, where I engaged in a substantial law practice. My clients benefited from the aggressive, competitive way in which I handled their business.

Every weekday morning I pulled my car out of the driveway punctually at seven-thirty to begin the thirty-three-mile trip to my office. Usually arriving by nine, I would sift through the morning mail and through telephone messages I had been unable to answer the previous day. After segregating the mail into groups, I neatly piled the corresponding office files on my desk. By 10 A.M. I was on the telephone, then hurriedly dictated letters, affidavits and other legal documents for the next hour or more. I always ate lunch between noon and 1 P.M. and customarily reserved the balance of the day for appointments, research, contracts, closings, etc. On mornings when I had to appear at a trial, I usually shifted my appointments and research to the evening hours. Most days I would leave the office between 8 and 9 P.M., carrying an attaché case crammed with the legal files and documents I wanted to review at home before retiring. I was too busy to engage in any physical exercises or sports all week.

Saturday or Sunday was reserved for my sudden burst of physical activity. In the summer I rose early and stripping to the waist, I mowed, fertilized, edged and trimmed the

16

lawn, spaded the flower and bush beds, and radiated with pleasure as the hot sun baked my naked torso and streams of sweat soaked my face and brow and eventually ran down over my body. During the winters I shoveled snow and painted and repaired the house.

Since I looked upon myself as being robust and healthy, I considered physical examinations unimportant, and rarely permitted doctors to examine or treat me. However, on reaching the age of thirty-nine, I reviewed my family history. My mother had died of a stroke at the age of sixty. My father, who is now sixty-five years old, had survived two severe heart attacks when he was forty-eight, and his younger brother had succumbed to a heart attack when he was forty-six.

Although I was an attorney and a reasonably intelligent person, I believed that what happened to my parents and uncle would not happen to me; and if it did, it would be a *fait accompli*. Foolishly reasoning that I could not prevent a heart attack, if there was to be one, I put my affairs in order by making a will and obtaining adequate medical, disability and life insurance.

If I had questioned medical men, read books about heart attacks and coronary disease, and secured information from national and local heart associations, I would have been able to recognize the symptoms which appeared in the next five years. I would have sought competent professional help, and perhaps prevented or delayed the stroke and heart attack that actually occurred. But like many people, I believed that by denying the truth about myself, I would continue to be in good health. Like many people, I wanted to believe that if I ignored tragedy, tragedy would pass me by. Unfortunately, the statistics weren't misleading. I was only fooling myself.

Coronary heart disease is the number one cause of death in the United States, accounting for 54 percent of the annual mortality rate. Making no distinctions, it victimizes the banker, doctor, lawyer, butcher, truckdriver, clerk or any other person. Compare it with cancer (which accounts for about 17 percent of all deaths and is the second leading cause of death in the United States) and you can easily understand why coronary heart disease has been called "Public Enemy Number One."

Tragically, though it kills approximately six hundred thousand Americans each year (almost one person every minute), coronary heart disease can be delayed and, perhaps, prevented, if the victim understands the conditions that cause it and seeks help. These potential victims (I was lucky) are predominantly men, frequently heads of households who are unexpectedly taken from their families at the prime of their productive years. Only Finland has a higher death rate from heart disease than the United States. Before coronary heart disease kills, it may cripple and disable its victims.

Males of all ages are much more at risk than females. Between thirty-five and forty-four years of age, five males have died from heart disease for every two females; between forty-five and fifty-four years, the mortality rate has been five males for every female; and twice as many men in their sixties or seventies have died from heart disease as women.

Statistically speaking, by the time the average American male reaches the age of sixty, he has about one chance in five of developing coronary heart disease. Furthermore, one out of every five men between the ages of forty-five and sixty-five can expect to have a heart attack within the next five years.

Fifty percent of all deaths from coronary heart disease

occur within the first twenty-four hours following the heart attack. Although many deaths occur within minutes or seconds following the heart attack, a number of these victims could have saved themselves either by adopting preventive measures earlier in their lives, or by recognizing the signs or symptoms warning of a future attack and getting medical help.

While about half of all heart attack victims die before they reach a hospital, of those persons who are fortunate enough to be hospitalized, approximately 15 percent die within the first seventy-two hours. Practically all survivors have a good chance of leading normal, active lives when they have recovered.

As I later discovered, men who have had heart attacks at a younger age are less apt to survive than men who have had the attack in the later years of their lives. Thus it was increasingly important for me to have begun preventive measures immediately upon discovering that I might be susceptible to heart attacks. Methods of prevention might have helped me either to delay the actual heart attack until later or to have avoided it altogether.

Attempts have been made to develop a character sketch of the coronary-prone individual, as follows.

The typical heart attack candidate appears to be about one or two inches shorter than his opposite number, while tending to be at least twenty or more pounds overweight in excess fat (adipose tissue) instead of muscle. He seems to smoke cigarettes and lead a rather sedentary life. Coming from families with relatively short life spans, he has had one or more close relatives who died from either a heart attack or a stroke. Additionally, he tends to have elevated blood pressure (hypertension) and high blood fats (lipids) such as cholesterols or triglycerides.

As a rule, he is ambitious and self-disciplined, a man who constantly works beyond his normal capacities. Appearing to be more compulsive, restless and aggressive than most, he does not usually manage his aggressive tendencies well. Gradually mounting tensions build up for months, even years, before the onset of the heart attack. He feels let down when his goals cannot be achieved, and though tending to work harder under increased stress and strain, he prefers to devote his efforts to solving mental problems rather than to physical work.

The common victim is unhappy and restless at home, and yearns to amass material possessions. He never stops to enjoy home life. Leisure time fails to yield satisfaction because he is too rigid and compulsive. A constant worrier, he permits stresses and strains to wear him down, but nevertheless presents a picture of serenity to the outside world. He has a tendency to repress anger and other emotions that might arouse hostility in others.

Only because of my knowledge of family history did I realize at the age of thirty-nine that I might possibly suffer a heart attack within the next decade. I didn't have the slightest idea of what statistical evidence was being compiled by the medical profession concerning persons who could be prone to coronary artery disease. I did not even have a working knowledge of the heart or the circulatory system, nor could I recognize the signs or symptoms of a diseased coronary artery or an impending heart attack. However, I seemed to be in excellent health, although I hadn't had a medical examination for a number of years.

Looking back, I can see that the first discernible signs of coronary artery disease appeared when I was forty. Not the classic dramatic signs of great pain, numbing of the arm or tingling sensations in my fingers, but barely perceptible indications which, nevertheless, were just as symptomatic. Moreover, my personality began slowly to change. Until then, I had been a fairly good-natured person, hardly ever short of temper. If a situation displeased me, I would be willing to discuss it calmly and effectively, and, at the least, consider the other person's point of view. The change was hardly noticeable at first, but gradually I became more and more irritable at home, lashing out at my wife, my children or anyone who caused my displeasure, not caring whom I hurt. So critical had I become about anything my wife would do or say that she bottled up her own emotions. When she suggested that we consult a marriage counselor, I shouted and raved at her and drove her from the house for several hours. Any innocuous word or action could displease me. The children started to shy away from me. My marriage, which had sailed so smoothly for the past seventeen years, had come upon turbulent seas and was about to founder on the rocky shores of separation and divorce. My wife often had to seek refuge with the children in her mother's home. We had become strangers in our own home; only our concern about the welfare of the children kept us together. I became a dual personality—one the seemingly placid person whom I tended to show to the outside world, and the other my real self, tense and irritable.

At the same time I noticed that I became breathless when exerting myself physically. It was not the kind of breathlessness that came from competing in sports or running great distances; instead I would start to breathe heavily when running up a flight of stairs (I had been able to run easily up two or three flights before) or when walking quickly up a hill.

I attributed this physical phenomenon to the fact that I had just turned forty and to the idea that with middle age, all bodily functions must necessarily slow down. Although this was not true, I preferred to rationalize rather than to suspect that something could be wrong. Two years later I experienced the first noticeable classic symptoms of coronary artery disease.

As usual that morning, I left my home at seven-thirty and drove in the bumper-to-bumper rush-hour traffic along the highways and city streets. Reaching my office a little past nine, I tossed the mail and telephone messages aside. Worried about an important case that I was to argue in court the next morning, I intended to spend the entire day in the office library, researching the law and reviewing the facts of the case. Inadvertently, my secretary had made an appointment for me with a new client at two o'clock that same afternoon. Not wanting to offend the prospective client, I was caught in a dilemma. Should I stay in the office and work through the lunch hour or work undisturbed in the relaxing atmosphere of some restaurant? I chose the latter. Leaving my office about noon, I planned to have cocktails and a leisurely lunch at a Chinese restaurant across town where, away from the stress and commotion of the office, I could review my notes.

Although the trip across town normally took only fifteen minutes, an accident delayed me. Concerned about the limited time I had in which to review my notes at lunch, I hopped the curb and sped down a side street, taking a different but longer route. Parking my car at the first available two-hour meter, I almost ran the three blocks to the restaurant. When I arrived, the place was crowded, and I had to gulp down my food.

Hurrying from the restaurant, I walked to my automobile, parked at the top of a hill. About midway, my breathing became heavy and labored; but I knew that the client would be waiting at my office and I struggled on. Then it happened.

As I continued, an invisible weight seemed to press against my chest just to the right of center. The pressure, almost centrally located at first, started to spread across both sides of my chest; I began gasping for air. My breathing became so labored that with each step I took I experienced a crushing and constricting sensation in my chest and lungs as though I were being squeezed in a vise. The struggle to breathe, combined with the strangling pressure across my entire chest and the accompanying pain in my lungs and throat, forced me to stop instantly. I felt as if I could not take another step without losing consciousness. For less than one minute I stood absolutely still. All signs of pressure, pain and breathlessness disappeared completely.

Not quite sure what had happened, I continued to walk to the car. There was no trace of the frightening phenomenon. In spite of the fact that my bodily functions had all returned to normal, I got into my car shaken and cursed quietly to myself. This was a new experience. As I sat behind the steering wheel, reflecting, before starting the motor, I cursed my secretary for making the appointment that had upset my entire day's schedule, the client for not accepting a later date, the accident, which had made me late, and the slow service at the restaurant, which had forced me to hurry with my meal. And as I again drove across town to return to my office, I concluded that gulping down that heavy meal, together with my worry about punctuality, had given me a momentary attack of indigestion. If it was anything else, the pressure, pain, constriction and breathlessness would still be there, or at the very least, would have returned. I was completely wrong.

What had just happened was the first classic sign that something was wrong with my coronary arteries. The pain and discomfort (angina pectoris) was the only way the heart muscle could tell me that it was not receiving enough oxygen; that one or more of the coronary arteries supplying blood to my heart muscle were not working to full capacity. If I had known all or some of this, I would not have blamed indigestion in so flippantly dismissing what had just occurred.

During the next eighteen months I had two or three similar experiences after eating heavy meals. They occurred at intervals of from three to six months and were never as intense as the first one. Each time the pain and constriction came, it would disappear after I stood absolutely motionless for less than one minute.

I refused to visit a physician. True, it was difficult for me to breathe when running or walking rapidly for any great distance; and I was constantly irritated and tense and desired to be by myself. But I attributed all that to middle age and mental strain, whether real or imaginary.

About this same time, I had a feeling of constant fatigue. No matter how early I would go to bed, on awaking I would be just as tired. As the months went by, I would arrive fatigued at my office. I was mentally alert, but physically exhausted and barely able to last through the day, drive

24

home, eat supper and go back to bed. All I wanted to do was to sleep, in the hope of somehow awakening refreshed. My legs felt as if weights were attached to them, and my shoulders and back as if I lifted heavy packages all day.

Reasoning that the tiredness also resulted from mental pressures, I planned to take a short vacation to some Caribbean island, far away from the demands of society. But my clients and their cases kept me too busy. I never took that vacation.

On Tuesday morning, the seventeenth of August, eighteen months after my first frightening experience, I was late in meeting one of my clients at the courthouse. Parking my car two blocks away, I grabbed my briefcase and hurried downhill. About halfway to the courthouse, I began to breathe heavily. That same feeling of pressure coupled with constriction crept across my chest. Stopping, I felt the sensation of pressure disappear, and I continued to walk a few more steps. But the pressure and breathlessness immediately returned, causing me to stand absolutely still for about two minutes. When I had reassured myself, I continued walking at an average pace.

Nothing further happened that day. The next day I again parked my car at the top of that same hill and hurried down at a fairly rapid rate. I had not walked more than a hundred paces when I became breathless and felt the familiar uncomfortable fullness about the chest. However, my business at the courthouse couldn't wait and I tried to go on.

After two or three more steps, it seemed as if an invisible force was slowly crushing the middle of my chest. I could not take one more breath without feeling unbearable pain. My left arm became so numb that I had to drop the briefcase in my left hand. For the first time in three years the pain would not go away when I stood perfectly still.

There was a building ledge nearby and I sat down, not daring to breathe heavily. I remained seated on that ledge for five minutes, while all signs of pain and discomfort disappeared completely and just as mysteriously as before. Reasoning that all I needed was a good rest, I resolved to take a vacation the very next week. Firmly gripping my briefcase again, I continued downhill to the courthouse.

The remainder of that day and the next were uneventful. As I continued to go about my normal routine, the experience of the past two mornings ceased to concern me. And as I drove to the airport to meet a client that night, I began to plan the vacation that my wife and I would take the following week.

A light rain started to fall over the city. Suddenly traffic slowed down practically to a halt. The heat, compounded by the heavy moisture in the air, made sitting in the closed car almost unbearable. Arriving at the airport twenty minutes late, I almost ran toward the terminal building. Just as I reached the doors, I was forced to stop and stand perfectly still.

The same disagreeable fullness about my chest, accompanied by difficulty in breathing, overcame me once more. I felt confused and frightened. My brow was covered with cold sweat and my breath became more labored. A feeling of nausea pervaded my body. I wanted to run, to flee from the airport. I yearned for the comforting safety of my home, family and bed. Abandoning my plans to meet anyone, I left a message at the airline counter that I was ill and would see my client the following day. Then I walked slowly back to my car and drove home. Upon reaching the house, I called to my wife. I had never told her about these peculiar physical incidents. But now I was shaken and frightened, weak and fatigued. I felt that I desperately needed someone to help me. I told my wife what had happened that evening. She became distraught. After making me promise I would call the doctor first thing the next morning, she got me undressed and into bed. Although I was exhausted, I could not sleep.

It had finally dawned upon me that something might be wrong with my heart. But, I reasoned to myself, how bad can it be? After all, these little spells just come and go. If I were really going to have a heart attack, I would faint and someone would call for an ambulance. Eventually I fell into an exhausted sleep.

The next morning I was awakened by the warm rays of sunlight through my curtained windows. Gone were all the fears, the pressures and the pains of yesterday. After taking a shower, I ate a leisurely breakfast and then telephoned the doctor's office for an appointment that morning. When I explained what had happened to me the night before, he told me to come to the office as soon as possible. Next I called my office and left instructions with my secretary. I consoled my wife by promising that I would telephone her immediately after the physical examination. Then I left the house.

As I swung onto the highway, I was rather carefree about the state of my health. Planning the vacation I would finally be taking, I wouldn't concede that anything could be wrong with me that could not be corrected with rest. I was blissfully ignorant about the near future and what it might bring.

2 THE DOCTOR'S EXAMINATION

Driving along the highway, I listened to the steady beating of my heart. It reassured me that all my tiredness, breathlessness and shortness of temper were the result of mental pressure only.

I had a strange feeling of contentment as I approached the doctor's office. I thought this examination was necessary only to reassure my wife.

I stepped into a large reception room and walked over to a window space, where I sat down and picked up a magazine.

A girl in white called my name and I followed her into a small, neat office. Framed certificates were affixed to a wall behind a desk, including two that attested that Martin F. Mines had been elected to both Phi Beta Kappa and Alpha Omega Alpha (the medical college honor society). Other certificates made it plain that Martin F. Mines had completed his internship, residency and specialization in a well-known hospital in New York City and was qualified to practice medicine in the state.

Dr. Mines came in. He was just shy of six feet tall; not slim, but lanky in build. He had a full brown head of hair, cut neither long nor short, and set off by gray sideburns. A concerned smile graced his lips. Marty and I had known each other for the past several years, during which we had both participated actively as committee members in a local scout troop. We had spent many evenings chatting with each other and had recently gone camping with the troop. I was glad I chose Marty.

Marty inquired about my wife's health and the scouting activities of my sons. I felt completely relaxed as he stepped back to his desk and opened the manila folder that had been placed there.

Dr. Mines proceeded to ask about the present condition of my health, the history of any childhood diseases and operations, the health of my parents, sisters and brothers, any physical or mental changes, and then about the episodes of constriction and pain, and what I thought they indicated. As I tried to answer the various questions put to me, he jotted down notes in the folder, his inquisitive eyes looking up to study my face. At last he told me to go into the adjacent examining room and get partially undressed.

Dr. Mines had been assessing both my personality and my psychological make-up. He was also judging my honesty and accuracy in describing my symptoms. Observing my general demeanor, he was able to discern many facts about my cardiovascular system and emotional temperament. For example, if my facial muscles were taut and knotted, he could judge that I was nervous and strained. If my facial muscles were relaxed and I appeared calm, he might judge that I was not only mentally relaxed but, in all likelihood, honestly assessing my own condition. If I had a worried expression, kept looking at my watch, talked unusually fast or fidgeted in my seat, he could get the impression that I was excited and emotionally upset and would have a high blood pressure reading.

In the examining room, a medical assistant measured my height and weight, noting any signs of obesity. She then took me into another room, where x-rays were taken of my chest cavity. The x-rays would reveal not only the position of my heart and its exact size and relationship to my heart cavity, but also some indication of the size of the individual heart chambers.

Back in the examining room, I was instructed to lie flat on my back on the examining table as she dabbed a jellied material on my legs, my arms and across the left side of my chest. A tiny metal plate set in a rubber belt was then strapped directly over each arm and leg where the jelly had been applied. Rubber suction cups with metal plates inserted in their centers were likewise placed over every dab of jelly on my chest. In turn, each metal plate was connected by a wire to a large machine standing beside the examining table.

She cautioned me to be completely relaxed while the machine was recording. The electrocardiograph was designed to pick up electrical impulses from the heart.

I felt no sensations at all. After flipping the switches to turn off the machine, the medical assistant removed the straps, suction cups and metal plates, cleaned off the jelly with gauze pads, cut a long roll of paper like ticker tape from the machine and left the room.

I was seated on the edge of the examining table, trying to figure out the meaning of all the wavy and zigzag lines that my heart had reproduced on the paper, when Dr. Mines walked into the room. After checking the electrocardiogram that had been produced by the electrocardiograph machine, he wrote something in the manila folder and stepped over to my side. Then he explained to me what the electrocardiogram was all about.

With every beat of my heart, tiny electrical impulses were sent out along the heart muscle, passing through my body in preset pathways, eventually reaching my skin. These electrical waves were produced in steady patterns, which changed in certain characteristic ways when the heart became damaged. Upon viewing these steady patterns, Dr. Mines was able to recognize both normal and abnormal situations, the abnormal situation and pattern differing for each disease of the heart. The visual reproduction of these electrical waves was called an electrocardiogram (EKG or ECG). The height and depth of the reproduced waves were compared by counting the horizontal lines on the paper, spaced exactly one millimeter apart. By counting the vertical lines, each representing 1/25 of a second, the duration of these waves was calculated. Thus, Dr. Mines was able to plot how the voltage of my heart varied with time as recorded in millivolts.

The wave patterns reproduced on the paper were similar to the diagram printed below.

The "P" wave was caused by the electrical impulses traveling through the atria, which are followed by the contraction of the muscles of both upper heart chambers. The "Q," "R" and "S" waves were caused by the electrical impulses going through the ventricular muscle, which are followed by the

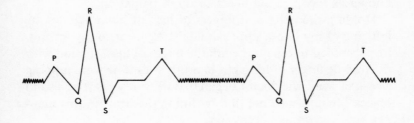

contraction of both lower chambers. The "T" wave represents the electrical recovery period of the ventricles and coincides with the mechanical completion of the heartbeat and the end of that particular contraction. Electrocardiograph phenomena are electrical and the "P," "Q," "R" and "S" waves actually preceded the mechanical beating of my heart.

The metal plates (electrodes) were placed on various parts of my body so that the electrical impulses of the heart could be measured and recorded as they traveled from one electrode to the other. The point between one electrode and another is called a lead, and each lead is recorded separately on the electrocardiogram and views the electrical impulses from a different angle or position. The direction of the impulse changes with various abnormalities. In turn, these areas of reference are labeled by specific letters and numbers (e.g., AVR, AVL, AVF 1, 2, 3; V 1, 2, 3, 4, 5, 6, etc.). In the reading of electrocardiograms, the position of the heart (i.e., vertical, semi-vertical, intermediate, etc.) is also important as a point of reference to the path that the electrical impulses follow from the pacemaker over the heart muscle.

Cautioning me to be silent, Dr. Mines put his hand flat against my chest. Repeating this at several different locations across my chest, he was able to locate my heart within approximate measurements. This method, I later learned, was known as locating the heart through palpation.

Holding the palm and fingers of his left hand against the left side of my chest, approximately adjacent to my armpit, he proceeded to tap on the middle finger of his left hand with the middle finger of his right hand. Just as if he were tapping a cask of wine, the doctor began to outline my heart as a solid object. He informed me that outlining the heart in this manner was known as percussion.

Dr. Mines started at a place far over on the left side of my chest, where he was certain that only the lungs lay. Shifting his hands in a straight line in the direction of the heart, he continued to tap in this manner until the sound that was heard changed from the hollow, drumlike thud of my air-filled lungs to the dull pitch of my dense, muscular heart. Dr. Mines then employed the same technique beginning from another position. By following several diagonal paths, he was able to gauge accurately where my heart lay, how big it was and how large an area it occupied in my chest cavity.

Next the doctor proceeded to take my blood pressure. What is measured is the pressure exerted by the blood against the walls of the arteries; and the pressure of blood in the arteries is produced by the beating of the heart. Each time the heart beats, the walls of the left lower chamber squeeze together, propelling the blood contained within it out of the chamber and streaming into the main artery (aorta). Because of the force with which the blood is thrust from the chamber, it flows through the main artery at considerable speed, estimated to be about three feet per second or 2.04 miles per hour, pushing and shoving onward the blood that is already there.

As a direct result of this forceful pressure at the mouth of the main artery, a pulse wave is sent throughout all the arteries in the body, directing them to either expand or contract to help relieve this great pressure and move the blood along. Since the walls of the arteries are made of flexible elastic muscle fibers, they easily respond to the pressure that is exerted with each beat of the heart.

A doctor can tell if a reading is low or normal, but he cannot judge whether a patient has high blood pressure (hypertension) if the reading is only slightly elevated until he has

33

read the blood pressure at various times, because an excited person can raise his own blood pressure.

Notating my blood pressure readings in the manila folder, Dr. Mines then set his stethoscope in both ears and placed the flat receiver over my heart. The stethoscope is just a means of transmitting the sounds of the heart while at the same time excluding all other noises; the receiver is actually a miniature amplifier. This method of listening through the stethoscope is known as auscultation.

Dr. Mines moved the receiver to various places over my chest, but always in the area where my heart was located. He informed me that if my heart were beating normally, he would hear only two sounds: *lubb-dub.* The rate of these two sounds, their rhythm, and even their pitch and intensity, have meanings. Most healthy, normal hearts make these two sounds. A damaged heart, diseased coronary arteries and diseased valves all sound different and their variations in rhythm, pitch and intensity mean diverse things to a doctor.

Putting his stethoscope back in his coat pocket, Dr. Mines then reached for an ophthalmoscope. The stem of this instrument contained batteries and the round head held a tiny bulb with a concentrated beam of light. All the lights in the room were turned out, and the doctor pointed the concentrated beam of light first at one of my opened eyes and then at the other.

Peering through the powerful magnifying lens, Dr. Mines was able to look into the back of my eye by concentrating the beam of light through the opening located in the center of the eye's pupil. By observing the condition of the artery blood vessels on the retina, he could form a further opinion about the state of my arteries.

Switching the lights on again, he next examined my mouth and nose, pushed his hands into my stomach to check the size of my liver and spleen, and felt for swollen glands under my armpits and over my neck. He also examined my throat, tonsils, teeth and ears. Next he tapped my elbows, wrists, knees and ankles with a small hammer to test the reflexes of my forearms, hands, legs and feet. He assured me that everything had a relationship to the heart and its functions, and that the whole of the patient had to be considered in order to rule out alternative causes of particular symptoms.

He then told me to get dressed and meet him in his office.

3 THE CORONARY CARE UNIT

In traversing those few feet between the examining room and the doctor's office, I was breaking through the barrier that separated conscious thought from the subconscious, the cushioned world of excuses from the world of naked truth. Still deluding myself about why I had come to be examined, I assumed an air of complete composure.

Dr. Mines was seated behind his desk, closely examining an electrocardiogram. He looked up at me and smiled. Settling myself into a chair opposite his desk, I looked at him questioningly. Marty's voice was calm, almost casual.

"Lou, on the basis of this examination, I feel that you should spend a few days in the hospital."

I was stunned and replied flippantly, "Sure, Marty, if you consider that necessary. I'll be taking a vacation next week anyhow." My head was starting to spin.

"I'll go home, prepare Hannah and the kids, and then I'll check into a hospital on Monday."

"No. I mean right now."

What he was saying to me was just starting to be absorbed. "You're the doctor, and if you think I should go into the hospital right now, I'll do it," I said. "A few days of rest wouldn't hurt me. But I have my car parked outside in the parking area. I'll drive home and have Hannah drive me to the hospital later."

"No, Lou! I will drive you to the hospital. Call Hannah and tell her to meet us there. As long as you agree, I will call now and reserve a bed for you in a hospital nearby that has a good coronary care unit."

My head was spinning furiously now. Obviously, I was more ill than I thought. "Coronary care unit" meant nothing to me at that particular moment. The only words that had registered kept repeating themselves over and over: "hospital" . . . "right now" . . . "a few days" . . .

Something was really wrong. Of that I was certain. But if it means only a short stay in the hospital, I thought by way of comfort, it can't be so serious.

After telephoning the hospital, Dr. Mines handed the phone to me.

"Tell Hannah what has happened. Then let me talk to her."

Like a robot, I dialed my number. On hearing my wife's comforting voice, my head cleared for a few moments.

"Hello, darling," I heard myself say softly. "I'm still at the doctor's office and I've had my physical examination. Marty suggested that I go into the hospital to rest for a few days and be treated. It isn't serious. Here—Marty's with me and he wants to talk to you."

My head was spinning again and I caught only the last phrase: ". . . so we'll meet you at the hospital in just a short while." Marty rose from his seat and stepped out of the room. Obediently I remained seated in the chair, my mind blanketed by a protective haze.

I did not know how long I remained seated. Then I became aware that Dr. Mines and two men were standing by my side.

"These are my associates," Dr. Mines was saying, "and

37

they will visit you at the hospital if I am unavailable at any time."

As I started to rise to acknowledge the introduction, Marty put a hand on my shoulder.

"No, Lou, don't get up!"

My God, I thought, what's this all about?

"They are familiar with your case and I want you to have full confidence in their capabilities. Of course, I'll be aware of everything that is taking place. But I want you to feel relaxed and assured if my colleagues ever have need to visit you."

That over, the other two doctors shook my hand and departed. I was so confused that neither their names nor their faces registered on my mind. My whole world seemed to be engulfed by a tidal wave of uncertainty, and I was drowning in it. Dr. Mines was the only thing I saw. His was the only voice I heard.

"It's time to go. My car is parked just outside the building. I've made all the necessary arrangements at the hospital. Your wife will meet us there later."

Silently I let him lead me past the little room containing the files and desks, through the reception room, which was crowded with other patients, out of the office, and out of the building itself. Once I was outside, the gentle August breeze seemed to clear my brain.

I realized that something was very definitely wrong and that I was being admitted to a hospital for a few days or perhaps a few weeks. But in my ignorance about coronary artery and heart disease, I could not know how extensive my condition actually was, nor what medical techniques were available to treat it.

In the car, Dr. Mines refrained from discussing the physical examination with me. Locked in his mind and in that manila folder in his office were the findings of the examination, which would be revealed to me only bit by bit. For he well knew that my attitude would be most important in effecting my cure. He had treated many heart patients over the years and knew that when I realized that my heart might be damaged and possibly stop altogether, I would be shocked and very fearful about the future.

What if I had objected to going to the hospital just then? How much would the doctor have had to disclose in order to shock me into the realization that immediate hospitalization was necessary? In my confused state of mind, how would I have reacted and adjusted to the worst possible news? And above all, how would my reactions have affected my heart condition and my life?

Wanting to avoid emotional conflict and shock, the doctor had used a "soft sell" approach to get my consent, and it had worked. The whole truth would be revealed to me when I was much better able to digest it.

Although the physical examination was essentially negative, disclosing nothing wrong with my organs, blood pressure, reflexes or heartbeat, a review of my personal history, confirmed by a reading of the electrocardiogram, revealed my condition. The electrocardiogram showed an elevation of the ST segment, and abnormalities in the "T" waves as well as with the "Q" waves in certain leads, which indicated that I had possibly suffered a past heart attack with resultant damage to the rear wall of my heart (a possible old inferior wall myocardial infarction). Lacking past electrocardiograms for comparison, it was difficult to ascertain when that damage had been sustained. Furthermore, the reading disclosed a flattening and inversion of the "T" wave in still other leads, which suggested that one of the coronary arteries had become so narrowed as to significantly diminish the flow of oxygen-carrying blood to a particular area of my heart muscle. My family or genetic history of vascular disease, which afflicted my mother, my father and his brother at relatively early stages of life, combined with my physical (height and weight) and emotional make-up, pointed to me as a definite "coronary-prone" candidate.

Tightness of the chest, pain and shortness of breath, particularly on walking after having eaten a heavy meal, were indicative of warning signals sent out by the heart muscle. These signals—angina pectoris—were the only way my heart muscle could cry out that the flow of blood through a particular artery had been reduced because that artery was partially blocked. Consequently, the supply of oxygen to the portion of my heart muscle that was being fed by that artery was not adequate for the muscle to properly perform its functions at that particular moment (coronary insufficiency). The heart muscle had to pump out enough blood, for example, not only to digest the heavy meal I had eaten, but also to perform the physical task of walking. Standing absolutely still for a brief time relieved my heart muscle of having to perform that double function, and consequently the tightness, pain and breathlessness disappeared.

Moreover, the recurrence of these symptoms, especially during the past few mornings, had confirmed the fact that I was experiencing a classic case of angina pectoris which was becoming progressively worse. My having had an attack of angina the evening before the physical examination had caused the doctor to be highly suspicious that my condition was becoming critical. This was substantiated by the electrocardiogram, which showed abnormal flattened and inverted "T" waves.

The finding of an old myocardial infarction (damage to the heart muscle wall) indicated that I had suffered a heart attack sometime in the past with relatively little damage (as measured by the size of the infarct) to my heart muscle. However, these findings could not tell the doctor when the attack occurred. It could have been anytime within the past several years, or the past several days, or the previous night. The personal history also disclosed that one of my coronary arteries was progressively becoming narrower. This was corroborated by the attacks of angina, which were occurring more and more frequently with less and less provocation. The flattening and inversion of the "T" wave (as shown on the electrocardiogram) signified that not enough oxygen (which is carried by the flow of blood through a coronary artery) was being delivered to a particular area of my heart muscle, that the flow of blood at that particular area was being slowed, and consequently that the artery was becoming progressively narrower.

After reviewing my personal history, as well as reading my electrocardiogram, Dr. Mines came to the conclusion that I was going to have a heart attack in the near future (an impending myocardial infarction) and that I would have to be hospitalized for observation immediately.

By insisting on immediate hospitalization in a good coronary care unit, Dr. Martin F. Mines undoubtedly saved my life.

The coronary care unit is a place where doctors, nurses

41

and technicians are immediately available. The purpose of the unit is to take care of the patient during the first seventy-two hours following the heart attack, considered to be the most crucial period.

The unit staff works on the assumption that death resulting from heart attack is not necessarily caused by the damage to the heart muscle, but can result from certain derangements in the rate or rhythm of the heartbeat, which can occur even where there is little damage to the heart muscle itself.

Dr. Mines stopped in front of the ambulance entrance. Asking me to wait, he disappeared into the hospital building. Two or three minutes later he reappeared, accompanied by a nurse pushing a wheelchair. Marty informed me that the nurse would take me to the coronary care unit, while he waited for my wife. I was taken in an elevator to the fourth floor and wheeled along a corridor and through a pair of swinging doors marked "CORONARY INTENSIVE CARE." Suddenly I could sense the intense battle for life that was being waged there.

To my right and left were three glass-partitioned rooms, each containing three beds. In the corridor between the rooms, two nurses were seated at a desk. Above it were nine small radar-style screens, across which flashed continuous electrocardiographic patterns. The scene reminded me of a television writer's conception of the control room of a space-ship—but this was happening to me!

From their desk, the nurses could simultaneously view all the patients and monitor their heartbeats. They worked quickly and quietly in the hushed atmosphere. I was to learn that these nurses were specially trained to read and interpret electrocardiograms, use all electrical equipment available in treating heart patients, and administer heartbeat-restorative drugs.

One of the nurses wheeled me to an empty bed in one of the glass-partitioned rooms. She gently reassured me that everything would go well, and I relaxed just a bit.

To overcome any objection that I might have about wearing a hospital gown instead of pajamas, she informed me that rapid recovery required as little strain upon my heart as possible. Any unnecessary tightness around my neck or waist caused by pajamas would force my heart to work that much harder to pump blood. This would impair easing the burden of the heart until the natural healing processes would have time to work. She said I could lie in any comfortable position, but warned me not to cross my legs, thereby hampering my circulation. I was to have complete physical and emotional rest.

Once again a jellied substance was applied to three or four places across my chest, over which were placed tiny electrodes, each secured to my chest by means of "pasties." Wires led from each of these tiny electrodes to an electronic system, situated at the head of my bed, which was monitored by special electrocardiograph monitors. Like Dr. Mines's electrocardiograph, these electrodes also picked up the electrical impulse waves sent out by my heart muscle. But instead of the waves being recorded on the specially ruled paper, here they were displayed on a luminous panel just above my bed (an oscilloscope), which coincided exactly with a duplicate panel, which I had seen in its central location at the nurses' station in the corridor just beyond the glass partition of my room.

Like radar screens, both panels continuously displayed luminous zigzag lines darting from left to right. These wavy lines, accompanied by a constant high-pitched sound of *beep-beep-beep-beep-beep,* were an exact audio-visual reproduction of the beating of my heart.

If the heart suddenly stopped beating, or started to beat wildly in an irregular pattern (ventricular fibrillation), a loud bell or buzzer would automatically be triggered in the monitoring system, alerting the doctors and nurses on duty to the particular emergency at hand. If the pattern shown on the luminous screen indicated that the heart was beating too slowly, or too quickly, or that the rate or rhythm became irregular, with multiple extra beats, corrective action would be instituted immediately.

This wonderful electronic device was substituting as a continuous electrocardiograph. And if a permanent record of a particular cycle was desired, a special device on the monitor enabled the medical staff to play back the last several seconds of the heartbeat, printing it on special ruled paper. All the patients in the coronary care unit were monitored in this manner twenty-four hours of each day.

Next, a flexible plastic tube, greenish in color, was looped behind my ears and under my chin. A branch, with two small nipples protruding from it, lay across my upper lip, and the nipples were inserted into my nostrils. The end of the plastic tube was connected to a large jar just above the head of my bed, which was half filled with bubbling water. In this manner, oxygen was administered to my nostrils in a slightly humidified condition. The nurse cautioned me to use the oxygen steadily in order to ease my breathing at the same time it relieved the burden on my heart.

Once I was relaxed, she took my blood pressure, pulse and temperature. Inserting a small needle into one of the veins in my left forearm (for intravenous feeding or I.V.), the nurse, in whom I had now placed my confidence, informed me that the head of the needle was capped with a spongy substance; and that the needle would continuously remain in place, enabling the doctors to inject instantaneously into the bloodstream any liquid or drug needed.

A white-coated laboratory technician arrived. He took a urine sample for analysis, and a blood smear from a needle puncture that he made at the tip of one of my fingers. Although these procedures were routine for any patient admitted into a hospital, for the heart patient admitted to the coronary care unit every act has a very special significance.

The sample of urine was necessary to ascertain whether or not there were any complications in the functioning of my kidneys, if I was a diabetic, or if my blood sugar was so high that I was in danger of developing diabetes. This precaution is necessary so that the patient will not be given the wrong drugs. The blood smear was to obtain a count of the white and red blood corpuscles. A high count of white corpuscles would primarily be indicative of internal infection.

He then inserted a needle attached to a hypodermic syringe into a vein in my right forearm, from which he withdrew five tubefuls of blood. These samples, taken daily, would be analyzed for levels of blood fats (lipids such as cholesterol and triglyceride) in my bloodstream. They would also be analyzed every day for enzymes produced by the death of any myocardial (heart muscle) tissue to note whether additional damage had been done. This is an added check on the electrocardiograms taken every day (serial tracings). Moreover, these samples would be analyzed for any changes in the sodium or potassium levels (chemicals mainly involved in the electrolytic beating of the heart). And the hospital laboratory would type my blood in case an emergency operation or transfusion had to be performed.

Another laboratory technician pushed a silent portable electrocardiograph machine to my bedside to take an electrocardiogram.

The technicians left. The nurses moved noiselessly through the unit. I looked at the machines, the white uniforms, the walls. What was I doing here? I lay apprehensively, awaiting the visit by Dr. Mines and my wife.

A half hour later they arrived. He said that all the hospital precautions were necessary because of the constricting attacks I had been experiencing; that I might or might not have a heart attack; but that if I did have it, the necessary equipment and trained personnel were available to me. He then turned to a passing nurse, issued some muffled instructions, told me that he would be visiting me every morning, and left. My wife and I were alone at last. No tears, no halting sniffles; she smiled sweetly, took my hand in both of hers and reaffirmed everything that Dr. Mines had just said. She also assured me that her mother would come to stay with her and the children as long as I was hospitalized and that she and the children would be cared for. Reassuring me that she would visit at every opportunity, she kissed my forehead gently and was gone. Immediately thereafter, a nurse stopped by my bedside and gave me a sleeping tablet, and I quickly drifted off.

That day my hospital progress record sheet read:

8/20   First admission of 44-year-old attorney because of
        recurring chest pains of four days' duration. Patient
        noted discomfort going into left arm associated with
        breathlessness when rushing for last few days and last
        night pain lingered, went into right arm. Today
        electrocardiogram shows T wave changes.
        Past history noncontributory.
        Blood Pressure 140/80; Pulse 80
        Ear, nose, throat—negative
        Lungs—clear
        Heart—regular, no murmurs
        Abdomen—soft
        Legs—negative [no hardening of arteries or veins,
        no inflammation of veins, normal pulsebeat over
        the ankles indicating sufficient circulation to the
        extremities, no muscular complications]

The electrocardiographic report read:

8/20   Intermediate heart. Deep Q wave in 3, smaller Q
        waves in 2, AVF. Slight ST elevation in V-2, 3. T
        wave inverted in V-1 through V-4, flat in V-5 and
        V-6. Nonspecific ST and T wave abnormalities.
        Possible old inferior wall M.I. [myocardial infarc-
        tion]. Old EKG would be useful for comparison.
        Serial EKGs [taken regularly every day] are in-
        dicated.

        Impression: Coronary insufficiency with impend-
        ing coronary.

                                                M.F.M.

4 THE HEART PATIENT

Death is no stranger to a coronary care unit. Between 70 and 80 percent of all patients who are admitted to the coronary care unit within those vital seventy-two hours following their attacks do survive, and for the most part, again lead normal lives. With advanced medical knowledge and discoveries, aided by a potential victim's recognition of the clues of coronary artery disease, death will eventually claim a significantly smaller percentage.

When I was in the coronary care unit the prescribed treatment for most of the patients consisted of physical and emotional rest, oxygen, anticoagulants to thin the blood, weight control by special low-calorie diets, and sedatives when necessary. Except in cases of extreme emergency, all treatment was designed to ease the work burden of the heart so that any damaged area could rapidly heal. All hearts were constantly monitored by electronic equipment for signs of abnormalities.

No telephones, radios or televisions were permitted. No equipment could be kept that would in any way interfere with the delicate electronic equipment in use. The nurses quietly checked each patient, gave prescribed medication and tended to their numerous other duties. Even in emergencies they never were excited, but quickly and silently administered to that particular patient routinely.

Only one visitor at a time was permitted to a patient. Visiting periods were restricted to fifteen minutes every two hours and limited to close relations. My wife was my most frequent visitor, not missing even one visiting period, and I felt assured that I had not been forgotten or completely cut off from the world outside. The wives, husbands, children and parents visiting the coronary care unit showed unusual concern for all the patients lying there. They would frequently smile, nod or wave to me when passing my bed. Every now and then, one would approach to ask if I was comfortable or wanted something. Sometimes they would walk up and down in the short hallway just beyond the glass partition of my room with solemn, expressionless faces, and I would know that their loved one, perhaps in one of the other rooms, had reached some crisis. Many of them would engage my wife in short conversations outside the room. They all shared a common bond—some loved one who was a heart patient in that unit.

I was immediately put on a low-calorie (about 1000–1200 daily) diet, with severely restricted salt intake. To digest large quantities of fatty foods, the stomach and digestive tract require an increased quantity of blood and the heart muscle has to respond by pumping with greater force and frequency. Salt tends to constrict the blood vessels, thereby forcing the heart to pump harder to push the same quantity of blood to all parts of the body through narrower tubes. Thus the ultimate goal of the diet is also to ease the work burden of the heart.

I was given heparin, an anticoagulant drug used to influence the clotting processes of the blood. These clotting factors are responsible for the formation of blood clots (thromboses) in the coronary arteries. Unfortunately, once a clot has already been formed in a coronary artery, there is no evidence that these drugs can dissolve the clot or limit its growth. However, anticoagulant drugs are used to prevent new clots from forming (especially in the leg veins) or to deter the fragmenting of existing blood clots. Of major concern is a possible breaking off and shifting of pieces of a clot from one place in the body to another. For example, the movement of a clot or a piece of a clot from the left lower heart chamber to the brain is almost always most serious; one traveling from a leg vein to a lung can prove fatal.

Heparin, the first drug I was given, is effective when injected through a vein directly into the bloodstream. Taken orally it is ineffective, because heparin is a chemical compound that cannot properly be absorbed through the digestive system. The coumarins, another group of anticoagulant drugs which I would eventually be given, are inefficient unless taken orally. Two principal drugs in this family, Dicumarol and Coumadin (produced in tablet form), were taken orally, then digested and finally ingested into the bloodstream. But as the heparin was able to be injected directly into my bloodstream, where it would work immediately, I was given injections of that drug every four to six hours during my first five days in the hospital. Following that period, Coumadin tablets were prescribed because they could be taken orally.

Except for one brief episode of slight chest pain, which occurred on the morning following my admittance to the hospital, my stay in the coronary care unit was without incident. That morning, an aide brought a basin containing hot water, soap and a washcloth, and set it down next to my bed. With the bed elevated into a sitting position, I began washing my body and felt a dull, mild ache in my chest. Fearing that the pain would intensify, I lay back on my pillow and pressed the buzzer for the nurse. In the few seconds that it took for her to arrive, the pain had completely vanished. After that episode, I was permitted to wash only my hands and face.

My heart was monitored and its beating was kept under constant surveillance every minute of each day; my blood pressure readings and pulsebeat were checked and recorded every two hours. Every morning, laboratory technicians would draw from three to five tubefuls of blood for analysis and would take an electrocardiogram. Also each morning, Dr. Mines would examine me, talk with the nurse on duty, check my chart records, compare the electrocardiogram tracings and examine the findings of the laboratory blood analyses.

There were no changes in the electrocardiograms, which had earlier confirmed the doctor's original opinion that one of my coronary arteries was partially blocked. He knew that in the usual course of events, either (1) the affected artery would become completely blocked and close off, the heart muscle area being supplied by that artery would become damaged (myocardial infarction), and I would have had a heart attack; or (2) I could suffer from the chest pains of angina pectoris for a short period, indicating that my coronary artery was only partially blocked, so that temporarily an inadequate amount of oxygen was supplied to my heart muscle area (coronary insufficiency), and then I could revert back to normality for an indefinite period in the future.

As of the fifth day, the electrocardiograms suggested that my coronary arteries were only partially blocked and that I could possibly live with this condition for an indefinite time. All physical examinations had shown that my blood pressure, pulse and internal organs were normal.

However, in view of my history, confirmed by the abnormal past electrocardiograms, Dr. Mines had decided to proceed with caution. If the chest pains of angina pectoris did not recur during the balance of my hospital stay, then I could be discharged with a condition of stable angina that could be controlled with medication. But if the electrocardiograph tracings were unstable, showing any future flattening or inversion of the "T" waves, indicative of a recurring coronary insufficiency, this could mean that a coronary artery was getting ready to close off completely. I was therefore transferred to a semiprivate room in the medical cardiac care portion of the hospital.

While my cholesterol level was normal, the blood samplings showed that I had an elevated triglyceride level. Taking necessary steps to correct this condition, Dr. Mines prescribed Atromid-S, a new medication.

The semiprivate room had two beds with a curtain divider between, two individual night stands, one telephone to be shared by the two patients, and a private lavatory with a sink and commode. My roommate, Carl, a man in his late sixties, was also recovering from prolonged attacks of angina. He was a pleasant chap and I enjoyed chatting with him about the topics of the day. However, he was mobile and due to be discharged soon, and I was still confined to bed. Although my visitors and telephone calls were restricted in order not to unduly arouse my emotions in any way, I would still see an occasional friend who had made his way past the elevator guard.

In the medical cardiac care wing, a number of practical nurses, nursing aides and orderlies assisted the registered nurses. For the most part, they were exceptionally friendly, courteous and capable. One orderly, Don, always advised me to "take it easy," "go slow," " do things slowly, but carefully"—and he was right. Like many other heart patients, I had a tendency to move quickly and do things vigorously. That was part of my personality and emotional make-up and perhaps a factor contributing to my coronary-prone character profile.

I was no longer given oxygen; my heartbeat was not being monitored, and I was now taking Coumadin tablets orally instead of being injected with heparin. The routine treatment was basically the same as that in the coronary care unit: physical and emotional rest and constant examinations.

My day would begin at 7 A.M., when a washbasin, soap, washcloth and towel were brought in by an orderly. I sat in bed and slowly washed and dried my head, face, hands and body. After I had completed combing my hair, brushing my teeth and shaving, the orderly would return with clean sheets. As soon as I was settled, the white-coated technician from the hospital laboratory would come to my bedside to withdraw four or five tubefuls of blood from an arm vein. Between 8:30 and 9 A.M., Dr. Mines would examine me, read and compare the electrocardiograph tracings, check my charts and prescribe medication. Finally, a breakfast tray would be put beside my bed.

Not long after breakfast, another laboratory technician would wheel a portable electrocardiograph machine to my bedside and take an electrocardiogram. Until noon I would peruse my mail, read, converse with my neighbor and sleep. After lunch I would usually read and sleep until visiting hours at 3 P.M. When visitors left at 5 P.M., supper would follow, after which I would again read or talk to my roommate until lights were turned out at 10 P.M.

All through the day, medications were given, blood pressures and pulsebeats were taken, and the orderlies and nursing aides gave alcohol back rubs to prevent me from getting bed sores. The watchwords were "Take it easy."

Of course, I was buoyed by the knowledge that the medical and disability insurance policies I had obtained several years before would pay for the hospital and doctor, as well as insure a weekly income for the family. And I was constantly in touch with my office through messages delivered and received by my wife and my father. Occasionally my partners would visit with me briefly, but I preferred not to discuss office problems with them in order to keep my emotions on a low level and not become aggravated.

Except for experiencing a slight twinge of chest pain on August 30 (ten days after being admitted to the coronary care unit), I was quite comfortable and, in my estimation, doing well. However, Dr. Mines would not permit me to get off the bed until well into the second week of hospitalization, and that was only to sit in a bedside chair. Blood-thinning Coumadin tablets were still being prescribed, as well as the Atromid-S to lower my blood triglyceride level.

Although I felt that the doctor was being overly cautious, I knew that he was the experienced physician and that I was his patient. After all, as an attorney I was accustomed to getting paid for giving advice. I also knew that when a client did not follow the advice I had prescribed, he usually made costly mistakes and regretted the result. I was determined not to make that error.

What I didn't know and couldn't realize was that my doctor's concern stemmed from his review of my entire picture, including the daily electrocardiograms. My personal and family history, coupled with my physical structure and personality, labeled me as prone to coronary artery disease. Moreover, the recent attacks of breathlessness and chest pain, which had brought me to the doctor's office, confirmed that at least one of my coronary arteries was partially blocked. Confirmation of that blockage was in the electrocardiograph tracing that Dr. Mines had made. Finally, a comparison of the electrocardiograms I had had taken since entering the hospital showed that a part of my heartbeat tracing (designated as the "T" wave) was constantly inverting itself and then reversing to normality. This condition (known as ischemia) was caused by an insufficient oxygen supply to a portion of my heart muscle. Another indication of ischemia is the depression of the ST segment.

Undoubtedly, I had a diseased coronary artery. But the doctor didn't know when, if ever, it would become completely blocked, damaging the affected heart muscle and resulting in a heart attack. For this reason Dr. Mines was being cautious.

The days dragged on. Although resolving to follow my doctor's advice unquestioningly, I became increasingly impatient. I wanted to flee from the hospital room and return to my wife, children, home and legal practice.

I was confined to my bed and room for the next ten days. The only privileges I had were to sit on the side of my bed with my feet dangling and to use the bathroom. Morning after morning I questioned Dr. Mines about allowing me to leave the hospital. Each day I became more obsessed with the idea of getting off the bed and out of the room. At last, afraid that I would become too emotionally disturbed, Dr. Mines permitted me to walk the length of the room to a big soft-cushioned chair, with the promise that I would shortly be able to walk in the halls.

That afternoon, I carefully slipped off the bed and stood on the floor in my bare feet. My toes tingled with excitement. As I took halting steps toward the other side of the room, I felt light-headed and dizzy. The floor did not seem to be level. Carl murmured words of encouragement. Holding on to the bed for support, first with one hand and then with the other, I walked slowly toward the big chair, about six feet away. I groped for Carl's bed and then held on to it in the same fashion as I had grasped my own. At last I reached the chair and plopped down into it. My strength was drained and I sat in that chair for about twenty minutes before attempting to walk back to my bed. I foolishly speculated that walking was a step toward getting me discharged and home. My hopes were short-lived.

Two days later, Carl was discharged and another patient was admitted to his bed. I can't remember his name. I know only that he was quite ill and I never got a chance to talk to him. That night he began to groan and call out loudly for the nurse. I pressed a button attached to my bed. The night nurse came to the room a few moments later, went to the groaning patient, talked to him in hushed tones, pulled the curtain around his bed and rushed out. Minutes later she returned with the resident medical doctor and his assistant. They stayed with him until the early hours of the morning. Despite the fact that I had taken a sedative, I was restless and the sounds of my new roommate groaning and the hospital staff attending him kept me awake most of the night. The next morning, I was irritable and couldn't overcome a sudden change in my personality. I could not think rationally, I was actually growling at the room, I wanted to scream at someone. It seemed as if I had drunk some potion during the night that had changed my character to that of a Mr. Hyde.

When my roommate started to groan again, I cursed and shouted at him. I began to throw my pillows about the room, and was suddenly gripped across the chest by an invisible giant hand, which started squeezing me until I became breathless. The constricting pain of angina had returned. Gasping for breath, I fell back across my bed, not daring to move even one finger. And as I lay absolutely still for a few moments, the giant hand seemed to relax its grip until it disappeared. I was so bewildered that I did not have the presence of mind to press the button for the nurse. An orderly was passing the doorway, and I called to him. Telling him what had just happened, he advised me to lie perfectly still while he called Dr. Mines, who was then in the hospital. I feared that this incident was a setback for me and I was right. Dr. Mines ordered an immediate electrocardiograph, revoked my walking privileges, and again had me confined to bed.

Consoling myself that this setback was only temporary, I hoped that if I did not become upset, I would once again be physically healthy. But the electrocardiogram taken that day showed otherwise. The hospital progress record sheet read:

9/8   No further pains.
      No fever.
      Blood Pressure 130/80
      Lungs—clear
      Heart—regular, no gallop, or rub
      Legs—Negative
      Electrocardiogram—"T" wave again inverted in
      right precardial leads
      Enzymes remain normal
      Pain undoubtedly an episode of coronary insuffi-
      ciency
      To obtain serial tracings

After conferring with Dr. Mines, that afternoon my wife
called a noted cardiologist to act as a consultant. The next
morning he reviewed the case with Dr. Mines, analyzed all
the hospital records and electrocardiograph tracings and reports, and physically examined me. He telephoned my wife
to say that he agreed with Marty's findings that I had experienced a heart attack before coming to the office, that the
channel in the frontal branch of my left coronary artery had
become narrower so as not to permit a sufficient supply of
blood to reach an area of my heart muscle, that there was a
possibility that the artery would stay open, and that the only
prescribed course of treatment was bed rest, anticoagulant
drugs and Atromid-S. Suppressing the detailed information
he gave my wife, he informed me that if I ever had similar
chest pains again, I should make an appointment to have my
heart and coronary arteries x-rayed by a fairly new technique
called angiocardiography, with the possibility of a coronary
artery by-pass graft through open-heart surgery. He left me

58

with the impression that the choice would be mine and that both procedures could be performed at my leisure. I was totally unaware that I had already experienced one heart attack and was on the verge of experiencing another.

The most recent chest pains and breathlessness of angina pectoris were signaling once again that something was wrong with my heart's supply system. Both doctors were of the opinion that this condition was caused by a severe narrowing of one of my major coronary arteries (atherosclerosis).

If chest pains continued, I would be in danger of having the artery become blocked and of succumbing to a heart attack, which could prove fatal. Modern surgical techniques are very successful in correcting this condition. If the chest pains should decrease in intensity and occur only when I indulged in a particularly demanding physical activity, then the condition could be controlled with medication; I would not be in any immediate danger of having a heart attack and surgery would not have to be considered until some future time, if ever. The doctors concluded that we should wait.

5 BACK TO THE CORONARY CARE UNIT

As I tossed and turned in my hospital bed—sleep was impossible—the pitch black of night imperceptibly advanced to pale gray, eventually yielding to the morning sun. The problems with which I had been wrestling all through the night, the uncertainty about my actual condition and what course to take, remained unsolved. I was concerned about the recurrence of the angina pain. What was wrong with my heart and coronary arteries? Why was I kept confined to bed? Why was I still taking the Atromid-S? Why did they keep taking electrocardiograms every day—and sometimes twice each day? Questions such as these, mingled with the fear of having a heart attack and dying, had troubled me throughout the night. Tense and tired from lack of sleep, I was unable to suppress a feeling of intense anger at my own ignorance that suddenly surged within me.

An orderly left a basin filled with warm water at my bedside, and I proceeded half-heartedly with the daily morning routine of washing, brushing my teeth and combing my hair. I was shaving when Dr. Mines poked his head through the doorway of my room to advise me that he was going to examine a patient next door. Continuing to shave, I resolved to question him that morning about my condition.

Slowly, a feeling of uneasiness overcame me. I started breathing heavily, as if I suddenly could not catch my breath.

60

A familiar pressing pain and discomfort crept over my chest, beginning just to the right of the breastbone in the vicinity of the fourth rib, as if heavy weights were being applied. Recognizing the symptoms from my other attacks of angina, I lay flat on my back, not daring to move.

Instead of stopping, the pain started to spread across the chest to both my right and my left arms. In desperation, I buzzed for the nurse and called out to an orderly passing my doorway to get the doctor. An invisible giant hand was squeezing my chest so tightly that I found it increasingly difficult to breathe. The pain spread across my back and, for the first time, I felt as if my back muscles were sprained. By the time Dr. Mines rushed into my room, followed by the nurse, I was writhing in extreme pain caused by what I imagined to be the twisting and knotting of the muscles across my entire back.

I tried to explain to the doctor that the pain was in my back and not in my chest. I cried out to him that my back was sprained and that all the muscles were knotting. After quickly slipping a small nitroglycerin tablet under my tongue, Dr. Mines gripped both of my shoulders with his hands and held me firmly on the bed, flat on my back.

When the nitroglycerin tablet had no apparent effect, he instructed the nurse standing by his side to inject a hypodermic syringe filled with Demerol, a synthetic pain killer (analgesic) and powerful sedative, directly into my left hip. Within seconds after I felt the slight prick of the hypodermic needle as it pushed its way into my hip, the pain subsided completely. The powerful drug had worked immediately, relaxing all the muscles in my body, and I was calm, serene and limp.

Instructing me not to talk just then, Dr. Mines took my

blood pressure and pulse reading; he left the nurse at my bedside while he stepped out of the room to order an electrocardiogram tracing of my heart and to make arrangements to move me back to the coronary care unit. I correctly assumed that the angina attack had seriously hampered any chances I might possibly have had of a quick recovery.

As in a nightmare, I vaguely recollected a white-coated laboratory technician wheeling a portable electrocardiograph machine to my bedside, an orderly assisted by the nurse removing me from the bed to a portable stretcher, and then being wheeled on that stretcher along the hospital corridors and back through the doors of the coronary care unit.

When I awoke, I was in another bed; the electrodes were again attached to my chest and sending out their transmittals of my heartbeat to an oscilloscope panel just above the head of my bed; the greenish-colored plastic tube containing life-giving oxygen once again encircled my head, the nipples jutting into my nostrils; an intravenous needle attached to my right forearm was connected to a tube through which dripped the clear liquid contents of a bottle hanging on a stand adjacent to my bed; and Dr. Mines was standing over me.

Explaining that I had experienced only another attack of angina pectoris, and that I had been transferred back to the coronary care unit just as a precautionary measure, Dr. Mines assured me that emotional relaxation and physical rest were the best treatment. He informed me that one of my coronary arteries was having difficulty in determining whether or not to stop working. Although this statement was truthful, it was a gross oversimplification of a complex problem. I was not sufficiently knowledgeable to question him any further.

I was put back on a liquid low-calorie diet. The doctor then whispered other instructions to one of the nurses, said he would see me the next morning, and left.

Upon returning to his office, I later learned, Dr. Mines consulted the cardiologist as to whether or not open-heart surgery would be indicated. He made an appointment to meet my wife later that day to bring her up to date on all the happenings, and to obtain her permission, should surgery be necessary.

Limp from the morning attack, I seemed to drift and doze through the balance of that day. Although my wife came to visit with me every two hours, she did not discuss the anginal attack, nor the consultations with the doctor. She did not display any fear about my condition. The nurse gave me a sedative that night, and though dispirited by the setback, I drifted off into deep, peaceful slumber.

The hospital progress sheet read as follows:

9/11   Patient had crushing chest pains this morning, spontaneously while sitting in bed. Color pale.
Blood Pressure 160/100; Pulse 80 regular, with occasional premature ventricular contractions.
Lungs—clear
Heart—good and regular
Abdomen—negative [no hardening of abdomen, no tumors, liver and spleen normal size]
Legs—negative
ECG—new depression of ST segments in anterior chest leads. To return to Coronary Care Unit.

Two electrocardiograms were taken that day, one immediately after the attack that morning, and the other several hours later. The respective electrocardiographic reports read as follows:

9/11   Semi-vertical heart. This is an abnormal EKG with nonspecific, but striking, ST and T wave abnormalities. Compared to the EKG of 9/9, the ST segment depressions are somewhat more prominent at present.

9/11   Semi-vertical heart. This is an abnormal EKG with nonspecific, but striking, ST and T wave abnormalities. Compared to the EKG done earlier on 9/11, there is less ST segment depression but increased ST segment elevation in AVF. However, on previous EKGs done earlier this month, the ST segment elevations were similar to present. However, if a Myocardial Infarction is suspected clinically, further serial EKGs are recommended.

The next morning I awoke refreshed and in no apparent distress. Once again I was able to think clearly and selfishly. I reasoned that yesterday's episode was just another of the attacks that I had been experiencing for these past years. What better proof existed than the fact that I had not had a heart attack and had felt no pain for the past twenty-four hours?

Actually, I had been mentally shaken and frightened by the violent nature of the attack. But since it had disappeared without leaving any noticeable signs, I felt that my condition was not too serious. I must be patient, hoping that my hospital stay would not last more than another few weeks.

Feeling more chipper than the day before, I washed my

hands and face, brushed my teeth and started gulping down my liquid breakfast. As I was drinking the orange juice, I was overcome by that same familiar sensation of uneasiness that had always presaged my attacks of angina. Pushing the breakfast stand away from my bed, I lay back and rang for the nurse. Within the few seconds that it took for her to reach my side, I was already experiencing the pressures across my chest and the breathlessness that accompanied my attacks of angina pectoris. Unlike the day before, the pains and discomfort were brief and were confined to my chest. I was frightened.

What did this new attack mean? Was I completely wrong about my prognosis? It was obvious that I was not getting any better, but was going downhill instead. That day I was too distraught to question either the doctor or my wife about what this new attack portended. By now my feeling of optimism had faded—but not quite to the point of pessimism.

In my ignorant state, I could not recognize the facts, understand the problem, or apply sufficient knowledge to the circumstances. This state of mind was new to me. Fearful of battling an unknown foe, I determined to hide my fears from the doctor and my family and endure to the best of my ability.

The rest of the day was uneventful, and I could do nothing more than read and sleep. Once I had resolved to fight my way out of this quagmire, I became reassured and calm. Hidden from me were the frustrations and fears of my wife and family. I did not know about the numerous meetings and phone calls that were occurring outside the hospital. Outwardly smiling and reassuring, my wife and my father, who were my only visitors, did not betray the hurried preparations that were being made at that time to have me transported to a large medical center for emergency heart surgery.

While washing my hands and face the next morning, I again experienced an anginal attack, similar in intensity to the one of the morning before, but not as severe as the attack that had sent me back to the coronary care unit. Since the attacks of angina were occurring steadily, with less and less physical activity to provoke them, I knew that my condition was becoming worse. However, as everyone wanted to spare me the anguish of knowing the gravity of my heart condition, I was unprepared for the emergency heart surgery that was going to be performed on the following day.

In spite of the sedatives given to me that night, I couldn't sleep. No one said anything that even hinted at what was in store for me in the morning. Perhaps it was just the sixth sense, which alerts human beings to some lurking imminent danger.

Having obtained permission from the night nurse to stay up late, I turned on my bed lamp and commenced reading a book, which kept my thoughts engrossed through the night and into the early hours of the morning. When I was awakened by a nurse on the morning shift, I realized that I was still wearing my eyeglasses. The opened book I had been reading was resting upon my chest.

After being washed, changed and fed, I endured the daily morning routine of having several tubefuls of blood drawn from one of my arms by a laboratory technician, having my blood pressure and pulse readings taken by one of the nurses, and having an electrocardiogram taken by another laboratory technician, who pushed about a mobile electrocardiograph machine. I was somewhat heartened by the fact that I had not experienced another attack of angina pectoris, and did not notice that Dr. Mines was unusually late in making his morning rounds.

When the doctor finally arrived two hours later, I was sitting in my bed engrossed in a book. Upon seeing him, my smile betrayed my confident attitude at not having had an attack that morning. I wanted to believe that I was finally overcoming whatever it was that had caused these attacks and placed me in the hospital. In response to my cheerfulness, Dr. Mines smiled back. On his lips was the same serious smile he had displayed in his office weeks before—that seemingly concerned smile which had portended the bad news that I would have to be hospitalized.

Carefully reviewing the history of my case with me, Marty Mines reminded me of the conversation I had had with the cardiologist on the ninth of September. He recalled to me that at the time we had all agreed to wait until I had experienced another attack of angina before being transferred to the medical center for angiocardiographic studies and possible surgery. Since my attack two days later, he had been in consultation with the cardiologist, and they had both concluded that I must be removed to the medical center at the earliest possible date. Then the bombshell was dropped —he was waiting for an ambulance to arrive, in which I would be transferred that very day.

My head started spinning wildly. The apprehension I had felt the night before was well founded. Weakened from my long hospital stay, the liquid diet, and the fears, tensions and doubts caused by the attacks, I could not speak. Just then my wife arrived.

Smiling cheerfully, she confirmed the fact that I would be removed by ambulance to the medical center that day. She indicated that this was the transfer for which we had all been hoping and waiting. Acting as though by this transfer my troubles would soon be over, she conveyed to me that I would soon be on the road to recovery.

What had never been related to me were the facts that since the first attack on September 11, I had been rapidly going downhill; that the situation was critical; that I was being transferred under emergency conditions; and that the doctors and surgeons were preparing to operate on my heart soon after I had arrived at the medical center. Had I been able to view the hospital progress sheet, I would have known the truth.

9/12   Few minimal pains since yesterday.
       Blood Pressure 100/70; Pulse 64
       Heart—regular sinus rhythm
       Abdomen—negative
       Legs—negative
       ECG—ST elevations now in 2 and 3 AVF
       STs slightly down in V-1 to 4 with marked T wave inversion.

9/13   Recurrent chest pains while washing.
       Blood Pressure 120/70; Pulse 80
       Lungs—clear
       Heart—regular
       Abdomen—negative
       Legs—negative
       Continues to have morning angina with ECG changes again today. Monitor shows ST depression at time of pains. Enzymes still normal.

9/14   Case reviewed with cardiologist. It was agreed that in view of the lack of evidence of through and through infarction and the daily changing ECGs, infarction is imminent. Patient is to be transferred to medical center for consideration of emergency coronary angiograph and consideration of by-pass surgery.

The electrocardiographic reports continued as follows:

9/12   Semi-vertical heart. This is an abnormal tracing with inverted T waves and depressed ST segment in V-1 to 4. The ST segment is elevated in 3, AVF. Compared to 9/11, there are no appreciable changes. Pulmonary infarction should be considered along with the diagnosis of arteriosclerotic heart disease.

9/13   Semi-vertical heart. This is an abnormal tracing with nonspecific ST and T wave abnormalities in 1, AVF and V-1 to 4. The ST segment is elevated in 3, AVF. Compared to 9/12, there are no appreciable changes.

9/14   Sinus rhythm. Semi-vertical heart. Diffuse ST and T wave abnormalities now involving leads 2, 3, AVF, V-5 and V-6 as well as the previously described leads. Nonspecific ST and T wave abnormalities are more diffuse than on the tracing 9/13.

One of the nurses came to my bedside. After depositing all my personal articles in a large brown paper bag, she handed them to my wife and asked her to step into the waiting room. Quietly and efficiently, she removed the intravenous needle and inserted a fresh needle into another vein in my left forearm. This done, she firmly and securely taped the needle onto my arm so that it could not accidentally be pulled out during the ambulance ride. Next, a sedative contained in a hypodermic syringe was injected into my buttocks. Within a few seconds, through a drowsy haze, I seemed to hear the nurse say to someone at her side that the sedation would keep me relaxed and calm during the transfer to the medical center.

Forcing my eyes to open, I saw Dr. Mines standing at my bedside holding my chart and talking to the nurse and two ambulance attendants. Noticing that I was awake, he said reassuringly that my wife would accompany me in the ambulance, while he would follow in his own car. Though the sedation had made me drowsy, I was awake and somewhat alert. As I was being wheeled out of the coronary care unit, I noticed Mary, an aide whom I had befriended, standing by the door. During the past few days I had been advising Mary about her marital problems. I had the attendants stop the stretcher for a moment. Trying to lift myself on my right elbow, I called to her not to forget the legal advice that I had given her the day before. As the stretcher was being wheeled through the doors into the hall, I wondered why she started to sob.

I was taken to the first floor, then outside the building. The stretcher in which I lay was lifted and placed in the back of the ambulance. My wife climbed in beside me, the doors were shut, and the ambulance rolled out of the hospital grounds, picking up speed as it reached the highway. Deeply engrossed in our own particular thoughts, neither of us said a word to break the uninterrupted wail of the siren as the ambulance sped along.

6 THE SHADOW OF DEATH

Situated on approximately fifty acres of choice suburban land, the well-endowed and well-equipped medical center was in a state of constant expansion. Its facilities included, among other things, a five-hundred-bed hospital, a nursing school, a newly equipped heart center, a fully staffed and equipped department of radiology, complete laboratory facilities, and an eminently qualified staff of physicians, as well as an association with a medical school which kept it supplied with promising young interns and residents. Interspersed among the buildings were large parking fields, numerous walks and carefully tended flower gardens grouped around modern sculpture.

But as I lay on the stretcher in the enclosed ambulance, completely engrossed in my own thoughts and fears, I was unaware of the medical center's location, facilities or grounds. My mind, numbed from the sedative, was unable to cope with my own immediate problems. I was not even aware of the dull pain being caused by the intravenous needle taped tightly to my left forearm.

I could not overcome the uneasy feeling of apprehension that now possessed me. Fear of the unknown had become my enemy. The accelerating attacks of angina augured that my condition, which had been serious, was now becoming grave.

Fear and ignorance were my worst enemies. I was fearful

about what would happen to me next, and almost totally ignorant about what treatment or results to expect. Within the next two days I would have to summon courage and help from whatever sources would be available to me in order to do battle with death.

But for almost total ignorance concerning my mysterious heart, I would have been able to discern under what emergency conditions I was then being transported. I would have known that open-heart surgery could save me from having a heart attack, with all its grave implications. And I would have been prepared for all that was to unfold within the next hour.

By the time I was carried through the emergency entrance for ambulance patients, and my stretcher had been set down on an ambulatory table just outside the corridor next to the emergency room, Dr. Mines had arrived. He had been following the ambulance in his car, and had hurried to my side. I owed a great deal of gratitude to Marty for his deep concern for me not only as a patient, but also as a friend.

He told me that since he was not an attending doctor of that medical center, I would be under the care of the cardiologist, with whom he would consult daily. Marty then gently placed one of his hands upon my right forearm and asked me how I was feeling. Although I did not know it at the time, the color of my complexion had turned ashen white, and Dr. Mines was quietly taking my pulse. He was fearful that I would have a heart attack at any minute. After the few moments it took for my wife to register me, I was whisked upstairs and wheeled through the doors of the intensive care unit.

The room was large and rectangular, almost like a hospital

ward unit. It contained eight beds spaced approximately three feet apart along two of the walls. At the far side of the room, parallel and adjacent to the wall on which the entrance door was placed, was a large desk, with a countertop above it, on which stood several telephones, pads, various instruments and files. This was the nurses' station, which, I later learned, was never manned by less than two nurses at any one time. On the wall behind was a large locked cabinet containing medications, solutions, sedatives and drugs. Above the cabinet was a white-faced electric clock with black numerals, hands and sweeping second hand, which would occupy my time and grateful attention for many of the days and nights to come.

As in the coronary care unit, on the wall next to each of the beds was an electronic machine with an oscilloscope panel, which measured and recorded the electrical impulse waves sent out by the heart. Also attached to the wall behind each bed was a jar of water from which those same green plastic tubes protruded to supply slightly humidified oxygen to the patient. Next to many of the beds were various other kinds of electrical equipment as well as plastic oxygen tents. Acting as wall dividers, which separated the beds, were white cloth curtains. All the patients and their equipment were visible from the nurses' station. Any sounds that were made in the room could be heard by the nurses as well as by each of the patients.

Only those patients considered to be most critical by the hospital staff were admitted to the intensive care unit. All open-heart surgery patients were brought there for the forty-eight to seventy-two hours immediately following the operation before being removed to a post-surgical-care floor. The

73

coronary care unit served as a secondary backup unit, into which many of those patients could be discharged.

As a patient's battle with death grew more difficult to win, the hospital staff had to rely more and more upon the victim's will to help with the struggle for survival. In order to achieve full cooperation, formal barriers between nurses and patients were removed. The nurses wore small identification plates pinned to their uniforms on which only their first names were inscribed. They were known to me as Pat and Sue, among others, and they always called me Lou.

For the most part, the nursing staff was young, under thirty years of age. They were all dedicated and had been intensively trained. They were kept hopping from critically ill patient to critically ill patient, administering sedatives, medicines and drugs, starting intravenous feedings, recognizing the various electrocardiograph readings that were flashed upon the oscilloscope screens, and assisting in the use of all of the complicated equipment, too numerous to mention.

During the day, at least four nurses were always on duty. In the evening hours, when most of the patients were given sedatives for the night, two nurses took care of the unit. In addition to the various attending staff doctors, a resident and an intern, who were assigned to particular cases, were always on call.

As soon as I was taken through the doors that led into the intensive care unit, a nurse called Pat came to my stretcher, introduced herself by name, and stated that she would be taking charge of me. Pat led the orderly wheeling the stretcher to a hospital bed located directly in front of the nurses' station, at the corner farthest from the doorway. Quickly and efficiently, she transferred me from the stretcher

74

into the bed and, just as efficiently, changed my hospital gown. Being in a corner, the bed had a solid wall acting as a divider on the right-hand side, and to ensure privacy, the cloth curtain was pulled completely around on the left side and across the front. Everything was very bewildering and I could not be absolutely certain of the sequence of events.

While Pat was drawing blood from both my arm and my finger, my wife popped into the curtained area, accompanied by my cardiologist and two other doctors. The cardiologist reminded me of our conversation the week before concerning angiocardiographic studies and possible surgery, explaining that in view of my worsening condition, the time had arrived to conduct these studies. He introduced the other two doctors as the surgical team who would perform the open-heart surgery if it was necessary.

He further clarified that I would not feel any pain during the entire procedure; that he was going to insert a small tube in the artery of my right thigh, shoot some liquid substance through the tube, which would outline my heart chambers and coronary arteries, and take x-ray pictures with special cameras that would tell him if one of my coronary arteries was being blocked; and that if one of the arteries was closing, he would alert the surgeons, who would immediately perform the operation. Informing me that he had to prepare the room and the staff where this x-ray cinematography would take place, the cardiologist departed and left me with my wife and the surgeons.

Assuring me that they had performed this "by-pass" operation many times, with phenomenal success, the surgeons carefully explained that they intended to remove a section of the large vein located on the inner side of my right thigh

75

(saphenous vein), sew one end to the main artery in my body (aorta), and sew the other end to the blocked coronary artery at a point beyond the blockage. They asked about my family history, as well as the personal history that had prefaced my visit to Dr. Mines's office. In the space of only ten minutes, I finally became cognizant that I was being prepared for open-heart surgery immediately following the angiocardiogram; that I had been rushed to the medical center as an emergency case; and that everything had been readied for this moment several days before. Naturally, I was bewildered and confused.

The two surgeons then excused themselves and accompanied my wife outside the curtained area around my bed. As they took leave of her, I heard one of them say assuringly, "When he comes up from the operating room, he will have numerous tubes sticking out all over him. Don't be frightened by this sight. It is necessary, and then he will soon recover."

Almost immediately thereafter, I had to reiterate my personal history to the cardiologist's staff, and then to the resident doctor who would follow my case, and finally to the intern who had been assigned to me.

When the intern had left, Pat entered with a urinal and requested a specimen of my urine. But the effects of the sedative with which I had been injected earlier that day had not completely worn off and though my bladder was filled, I could not urinate voluntarily. I knew that the hospital laboratory had to have that specimen before I could be anesthetized, in order to determine the sugar and acid content of my body for the operative procedures that were to follow. However, try as I could, I was not able just then to voluntarily control the muscles of my bladder.

After about ten minutes had passed without any positive results, the intern reappeared carrying a long, thin plastic tube, a plastic bag and some other equipment wrapped in a towel. After informing me that they could wait no longer for the urine specimen, he proceeded to catheterize me. Coating the end of the plastic tube with a specially treated jelly, he pushed it through the opening of my penis until it reached my bladder. As soon as the tube was inserted into my bladder, the urine drained out completely into the plastic bag.

Before I had been able to recover from the shock, discomfort and burning sensation of pain all along my penis and urinary tract—the tube had not been removed—I was visited by an orderly carrying a double-edged safety razor and a basin filled with warm soapy water. Explaining that he had been instructed to prepare my body for the operation, he proceeded to shave all the hair from my chest, abdomen, pubic area and right thigh. After the orderly had finished his job and departed, I lay back on my pillow, thoroughly exhausted and somewhat panic-stricken.

The pain and burning sensation in my penis and bladder had not subsided; the intravenous needle that was still taped tightly to my left forearm burned and stung me; my constitution was weakened by nearly three and a half weeks of hospitalization and dieting; and I was not mentally prepared for the unknown operative procedures that I now had to endure. Summoning all the courage I could muster under those circumstances, I resolved to fight any fears that possessed me, whether real or imaginary, in order to survive.

I was just beginning to feel more at ease when Pat entered and withdrew the curtained divider from around my bed. Directing me to lie back quietly, she began to push the bed across the room toward the doors. Until that time I was unaware that all the beds in the intensive care unit were mounted on wheels.

Pat easily manipulated the mobile bed through the doors, along the corridors and into the elevator, while simultaneously talking to me to relieve my tensions. But upon leaving intensive care I was suddenly overwhelmed by apprehension that something was going to happen that would interfere with the operative procedures.

I have never been able to explain logically my feeling at that moment, except to say that most people, at one time or another, know that an inexplicable event is going to alter the pattern of their life. It was not a sense of death, but rather the realization that an unknown factor was going to intercede which would prevent the planned operation from being completed.

As I was being wheeled into the room where the angiocardiographic studies were to be conducted, Pat's last-minute instructions were, "I'll be with you when you come up from the operating room. Be sure to cough from the stomach three times, even if it hurts, and then you'll be fine."

The room was moderately large, perhaps about three hundred square feet. On the far wall, opposite the doorway through which I had entered, were television screens, panels, gauges, meters and electrical switches of varied types, sizes and shapes. Directly in front of the paneled wall stood a large examining table, usually associated with the taking of x-rays, over which were hung, either from the ceiling or bracketed from the paneled wall, amphitheater lights and several different kinds of x-ray camera. Levers and buttons controlled the movements of the table, which could be raised and lowered, and tilted at any angle from head to toe or from side to side.

Many other pieces of electrical equipment of the latest type, which could be used in case any emergency situation developed during the course of the angiocardiographic procedure, were also at hand and in the room.

Removing me from my bed, two radiological technicians transferred me carefully to the huge table, placed a pillow under my head, and fastened my body securely with thick leather belts. The cardiologist then introduced the rest of the medical team, which included a radiologist, an anesthetist, an assisting nurse and several assisting members of his own staff. Each of them was garbed in a green surgical gown, hat and facial mask.

Although I was still physically uncomfortable because of the intravenous needle taped too tightly to my left forearm, and the burning sensation of the catheter tube inserted into my bladder through my penis, I was mentally at ease. I knew that I had nothing to fear but fear itself. The cardiologist then explained all that would be happening to me.

During the entire procedure my heart would be monitored, as well as my blood pressure and pulsebeat. In order to keep me awake and alert at all times, I was going to be injected with a local anesthetic, Novocaine. The large artery in my right thigh (right femoral artery) would be punctured and a tiny catheter tube would be inserted in it along a guide wire until the tube reached the arteries that fed my heart (coronary arteries). The guide wire would then be removed in favor of a harmless radiopaque liquid dye which would be inserted through the catheter into my coronary arteries and into the heart chambers. By this means, x-ray visualization of my coronary arteries and heart chambers would be permitted. All the while, both motion and still pictures were to be taken by means of specially developed x-ray cameras located above and below the table. For short periods of time, I was going to be subjected to intense heat while the x-ray motion pictures were taken. All that I had to do was lie back as comfortably as possible and try not to move.

My vision of the doctors and their equipment was obstructed by a cloth shield that was placed across the upper portion of my chest, from shoulder to shoulder. Beginning his step-by-step explanation of the procedure, the cardiologist said that I would feel a slight prick as he inserted the hypodermic needle containing the Novocaine into my right upper thigh. As he said this, I did feel a slight prick, followed by a sensation of numbness throughout my entire body. He next stated that I would feel a pressure in the vicinity of my right upper thigh as the artery was being punctured. As soon as I felt an enormous pressure in that area, his calm voice seemed to be saying that the artery was punctured, they were inserting the guide wire and catheter, and that I should just lie back and tell him when I felt uncomfortable during the remainder of the operative procedure.

At the direction of the cardiologist, the x-ray technicians started to raise, lower and tilt the table into various angular positions as the guide wire and catheter wended their way through my arteries and closer and closer to my heart. Suddenly I was subjected to intense heat caused by the flood lamps as the motion pictures started. I began to perspire and my body seemed to slide forward and backward on the movable table.

The heat was becoming unbearable when I noticed a numbing, prickly sensation in my right hand and forearm. The numbing sensation was traveling up my arm toward my right shoulder. I tried to call out to the x-ray technicians, to the doctors, to anybody—but to no avail. As if I were deep in the throes of a nightmare, no sounds could issue from my throat. I could not utter even one syllable. By the time that this numbing had reached my right shoulder, I was sinking into a swirling sea of blackness. I heard the nurse calling out, "He's going into—" and then I was unable to hear anything else as I was cast into a darkness filled with shopping carts from which unknown wares were being sold—and then total blackness.

Then I heard my name being called repeatedly and felt my face being gently slapped by one of the staff doctors. Upon opening my eyes, I saw the doctor with his face very close to mine. I couldn't utter any sounds nor lift either my right hand or right foot. Following his directions, I shook my head in response to his questions before again sinking into that sea of blackness.

During the course of the operative procedure, my heart had developed an extra heartbeat (extrasystole), which was not of itself uncommon; it may even be found in normal hearts. But as the doctors proceeded to insert the catheter, I had a stroke (left hemispheric lesion), which paralyzed the entire right side of my face, my right limbs and extremities. Almost instantaneously, my heart started racing wildly in an uncontrolled quivering which finally developed into a mass of writhing muscles, working without any purpose or effect and ceasing to pump the blood out into my body or brain (ventricular fibrillation). Unless this condition was corrected within one or two minutes, death would have been inevitable.

To meet just such an emergency, one of the electrical machines available to the medical team was an apparatus

81

that could electrically shock my heart and correct the disordered rate and rhythm of my heartbeat. This wonderful machine (defibrillator) had a pair of wires with metal paddles (leads), which were placed over either side of my chest, just above my heart. A switch located on one of the paddles was flipped, sending an electrical current through my heart. The electrical jolt, which sounded like a giant fist pounding on my chest, made my unconscious and somewhat lifeless body jump into the air. This electric shock, passing through my body for an infinitesimally short period of time, had the effect of stopping the heartbeat for one instant so that when my heart started to beat again, the heart muscle fibers, which instead of acting in a concerted sequential pattern with one another were contracting independently of each other in no particular rhythm, would become synchronized into a normal pattern. This procedure, known as polarizing the electronic field across the heart, actually restored my unconscious form to the world of the living.

I opened my eyes slowly to find that I was again in the hospital bed and back in the intensive care unit. Through the foggy mist that clouded my brain, I seemed to distinguish the form of my wife bending over me. Trying to speak, I discovered that no sounds would issue from either my lips or my throat. Although I was thirsty, I could not swallow.

Adding to my total discomfort were the tape wound too tightly around my left forearm to secure the intravenous needle; the burning sensation of the catheter inserted into my penis; a constant dull pain in the area of my right groin, where the artery had been punctured; and the heavy weight of a miniature sandbag pressing against my right groin. The blood spurts upward from the punctured artery and when the puncture is made large enough to accommodate a catheter, heavy pressure must be applied for a period of several hours to make certain that the blood will clot and close the wound. The sandbag placed on top of the sterile dressing ensured this pressure directly over the wound. Green plastic tubes bringing humidified oxygen again encircled my head, with their nipples jutting once more into my nostrils. Wires were again secured to my chest by means of "pasties," and the oscilloscope screen above the head of my bed continued constantly to record the electrical impulses of my heart beats.

One by one the doctors came to my bedside, in descending order of their importance in the hierarchy of the medical center, each testing the reflexes of my right leg and arm, the grip of my right hand, and my gag reflexes. First to arrive was the cardiologist, accompanied by the heart surgeons; then came the cardiologist's staff, next the resident in charge of my case, and last the lowly intern who had been assigned to me. In response to my glances and the shaking of my head, each one separately assured me that my vocal disability was temporary and that I would be able to swallow and speak within the next few days.

However, on overhearing the cardiologist's conversation with my wife, I learned that a stroke had occurred before the angiocardiographic study could be started and that both the study and the operation had been postponed.

Did I have a stroke or did I just faint? Either alternative was too much for me to bear at that moment. Coupled with a feeling of inadequacy from losing control during the operative procedure was the fear that I might have to endure the pain and misery all over again, but this time without the use of my voice and lacking the ability to swallow. In a moment I was gratefully engulfed in the sea of blackness.

7 DEPTHS OF DESPAIR

Since the open-heart surgery could not be performed, I was treated as a patient who could have a heart attack at any moment (acute myocardial infarction). Because of the stroke and ventricular fibrillation that had occurred during the angiocardiographic studies, as well as my poor physical condition, it was feared that the damage (infarct) to the heart muscle would be quite severe and that the attack when it came could prove fatal. Consequently, I was kept in the intensive care unit, where I could remain under the constant supervision of the medical and nursing staff.

I remained in a twilight world of forced dreams, not fully awake or asleep, and not quite aware of where I actually was or what would eventually happen to me. Although the cobwebs were slowly being swept from my brain, I could not seem to move my pain-racked body. My vision was blurred and my right limbs would not respond.

I became conscious that I was not experiencing some nightmare that would soon vanish with the dawn, but that I was alone, in a hospital and in some distress. And despite the fact that a curtain had been partially drawn around my bed, I could distinctly hear all sounds being made in that dimly lit room.

Sometime during that night, I was suddenly awakened by

the sound of excited voices accompanied by several pairs of feet scurrying across the room. My heart started beating faster and faster as I seemed to sense the intensity of an emergency situation that was happening close by.

A female voice (which I assumed to belong to one of the nurses) called out, "He's going into ventricular fibrillation. Hurry with the defibrillator!"

After several seconds had elapsed, a male voice warned, "Put that paddle over here. Good! Now, everybody get off the bed!"

This command was followed immediately by a very loud thud, as if one of the doctors had sent his clenched fist crashing down upon the patient's chest. This drama was repeated over again and concluded with that same sickening thud.

Then someone said, "It's all over. He didn't make it." And I heard the sounds of the doctors, nurses and equipment quickly moving away—followed by that silence which always settles over a hospital ward during the night.

Horrified by the imaginary vision of a strapping doctor pounding with his clenched fists upon some helpless victim's chest until, at last, he died, I silently prayed that neither my sons nor my daughters would ever enter the medical profession, with its power to decree life or death for some unfortunate patient. Then I slipped again into the sedated world of semiconsciousness.

How could I have realized at the time how unfair my attitude was toward the medical staff then on duty? These young doctors and nurses had to battle each day to save the lives of patients in the intensive care unit. And sometimes they lost. But more often they would be able to snatch the intended victim from the jaws of death. They were truly dedicated, devoted and remarkably well-trained young people who performed their duties to the utmost of their capabilities. In the awful days that followed, I learned to appreciate them fully.

When I next awoke, I noticed that the drowsy protective haze had finally cleared from my brain and that I was no longer under the influence of sedatives. Glancing around, I realized where I was and for what purpose I had come to the hospital. As I listened to the rhythmic *beep-beep-beep-beep-beep* of the monitor just above my bed, I also became aware of a tightening feeling gradually creeping across my chest. Although I tried to call to one of the nurses on duty, my lips would not move and no sounds issued from my throat.

By now the tightening sensation was accompanied by the pressure of a heavy weight against my chest and my breathing became labored. Unable to move my right arm, I attempted to attract attention to myself by slightly waving the left arm, into which the intravenous needle was inserted. And as if in response to the panic that was welling up inside me, a nurse called Sue appeared at my bedside.

Shaking my head in the affirmative to her question of whether I was in pain, she quickly went to the cabinet behind the nurses' station and returned with a hypodermic syringe and needle. I was breathing heavily because of the unbearable pressure on my chest, but Sue assured me that I was not having a heart attack just then and that the Demerol she was going to inject me with would make all the pressure and pain disappear.

Since returning to my bed in the intensive care unit, I had been lying flat on my back with the sandbag pressing upon my right groin. Explaining that she did not want to change my position and that she could not inject the needle into either my right limbs or side (which were paralyzed) or my left arm (which already had the intravenous needle inserted into it), she gently bent my left leg, injected the hypodermic needle into the calf, and lowered it again. Placing her hand upon my forehead, she calmed my fears by assuring me that she would not leave my side until I was asleep.

Within seconds, the pain and pressure had completely disappeared as a wave of numbness passed through my body. The powerful drug had taken effect and I lapsed into a coma-like sleep. Until I would have my heart attack, I experienced the constant attacks of angina pectoris during most of my waking moments. These attacks came without any apparent provocation and disappeared just as quickly when I was injected with Demerol.

Working on the midnight to 8 A.M. shift and going to school during the day, Sue was born to be a nurse. Perhaps twenty or twenty-one years of age, she was emotionally mature beyond her years; she was a natural mother to all patients, regardless of their age. She went through the intensive care unit every night, and with her soft voice and gentle ways eased the pains and calmed the fears of the troubled patients lying there.

I awoke to see the first rays of light creeping into the room. Approaching my bedside with a pleasant smile upon her lips, Sue inserted a fresh intravenous needle into my left forearm and removed the sandbag. Trying to make me feel more comfortable, she washed my hands and face and changed the position of my body so that I lay upon my left side. And for the first time, I fully realized what had happened to me.

I discovered that I could not talk, swallow, smile or even open my lips. If I could have viewed myself in a mirror just then, I would have been severely shocked to learn that the entire right side of my face was grotesquely twisted out of shape. I could not eat or drink and was nourished solely through the intravenous needle.

Testing my right limbs, I was happy to learn that I could manipulate my right leg; that I was able to move my right forearm, arm and shoulder; and that although my grip was weak, I was able to use my right hand. Despite the fact that the vision of my right eye was still blurred, the thought that I would be able to communicate in writing encouraged me.

While making morning rounds, the cardiologist and his staff stopped by my bedside. I was told that I had experienced a minor stroke while being examined, but that my muscles and reflexes would return to normal within a few days. Indeed, my right limbs were already recovering. But I was mostly concerned with my being unable to talk or swallow. How would this affect my future life and livelihood? And even if I eventually regained the use of my throat muscles in swallowing, would I ever be able fully to recover my speech? I was despondent, plagued by these doubts and fears.

It was one thing to know that I was shortly to have a heart attack—I would either recover or die, and although this prospect in itself was frightening, I could cope with the situation by rationalizing that I was in an emergency unit of the hospital with all its specially trained staff, its latest equipment and the most modern techniques available. (I didn't know then that my inevitable heart attack was expected by many to be fatal.)

But the thought that I might have to live the remainder

of my life as a vegetable, or with some permanent disability, unhinged me. What would I do to support my family? My speech was a vital factor in the earning of my livelihood. Even if I would never address another court or jury, I would still have to speak to my clients as well as to other attorneys. These questions haunted me.

Weakened from weeks of hospitalization and dieting, further debilitated by the rigors of the uncompleted angiocardiographic study, the ventricular fibrillation and the stroke, I was unable to master my emotions and wept. If it were only a heart attack, from which I would recover, I would probably be able to retain my physical as well as my mental powers even though I might have to alter some of my habits. A stroke, however, was an entirely different situation.

The stroke had caused damage to a portion of the left side of my brain (left hemispheric lesion), which had affected the right side of my body (right hemiparesis with right facial palsy and dysphagia). If the stroke was indeed minor, I would be able to regain the near normal use of my mind and body. But if my stroke was severe, I could be incapacitated for the rest of my life by the complete loss of my speech— or worse. And if I had to undergo rehabilitation, it might be many long weary months before I would be able to almost function normally, if ever.

I was very depressed and wept silently most of the time. As I lay in bed like a vegetable, only my brain was active. Thank God that my mind wasn't gone also! I thought about my past life—my school days, my marriage, the birth of each of our children, the years of building my law practice, and of how happy my wife and I had been in our home. I panicked when I thought about not recovering from the stroke.

How would I live? My home and my practice would be gone. I would not be employable. God, I didn't want to be a freak and a liability, dependent on my wife and the charity of the world for the rest of my life. During the intervals in which I was awake and lucid, I often thought that the only solution to my problems would be death. However, these intervals were short-lived, for whenever I was awake and lucid, I would have the pain and pressure of angina, accompanied by breathlessness, I would again be injected with Demerol, and lapse into semiconsciousness. Whenever I had these attacks, I attracted attention by tapping with a metal cup against an iron railing along the side of my bed.

Visitors were allowed to stay for only ten minutes every two hours. Every time I would have a semi-lucid interval, my wife and my father were at my bedside. Keeping a large yellow pad and pencil handy, I tried to communicate my thoughts in writing. I couldn't think in complete thoughts or sentences, only in individual words (e.g., "pain" . . . "chest" . . . "how" . . . "children" . . . "sedative"), and quite often I would misspell even those simple words. They were key words, and my wife and father seemed to understand and responded verbally. Because of my state, the lack of muscular coordination in my right hand and arm, and the blurred vision of my right eye, I could only print slanting letters that measured about three to four inches in height. But I was satisfied that at least I could communicate my thoughts to people and that they could reply.

I was completely unaware of time. Each second seemed like a minute, each minute like an hour, and each hour like a day. In my semiconscious state there was no day and no night, just the endless infinity of time, time in which I lay on

90

my bed in constant pain and discomfort, weak from lack of food, and listening to the loud, never-ending *beep-beep-beep-beep-beep* of the monitor.

I had been in the medical center for only one and a half days, but it seemed as though many weeks or even months had passed. The ambulance had arrived about one o'clock in the afternoon on Tuesday, September 14, and it was then only Wednesday, September 15, about 10 P.M. I was lying in my bed half awake when I began to feel those same agonizing pressures and pains across my chest. Somehow this time they seemed to be more intense. I started to bang frantically with my cup on the iron bed railing to attract the attention of the medical staff.

The resident assigned to my case glanced quickly at the monitor that was registering my heartbeat and then ordered a nurse to bring a hypodermic syringe and needle. Judging from the expression on his face, I knew that this was no ordinary attack, but one that was close to the anticipated fatal heart attack.

The pain and constriction of an angina attack indicate that an area of the heart muscle is not being sufficiently supplied with oxygenated blood. It may or may not register on the monitor screen or in an electrocardiogram; however, if it does register, angina can be noted as a depressed ST segment, an inverted "T" wave, or both. Angina culminates in a heart attack when the coronary artery becomes completely blocked, entirely cutting the blood supply to that area, which causes the muscle tissue cells to die (infarction). The death of these tissues registers as an elevation of the ST segment together with a "Q" wave. When the scar tissue finally forms, there is a deepening of the "Q" wave.

91

After ordering another nurse to bring a portable electrocardiograph machine to my bedside, the resident himself injected the Demerol directly into my buttocks. As my body grew numbed and limp, he secured the tiny metal plates of the electrocardiograph to my feet, arms and chest and took a reading. Before I was able to drift off into a sedated slumber, he had unhooked the electrodes, wheeled the machine away from my bedside, and walked calmly out of the room. I complimented myself for guessing that although the angina attack was unusually strong, it was not the expected heart attack. Slipping once more into that protective darkness, I was not aware that this attack was but the prelude to the battle in which I would eventually be engaged with death itself. The prelude is only the angina pain brought on by the narrowing of the artery and an insufficient flow of oxygenated blood to an area of the heart muscle. This is a wound from which the cells cannot regenerate, and can only be covered over with scar tissue.

It was the middle of the night by the time I opened my eyes again. Long shadows were cast upon the wall behind the nurses' desk, where Sue, the night nurse, was seated, working by the light of a shaded lamp. Except for the constant *beep-beep-beep-beep-beep* of the monitors in the room, there was no sound. It was then that I silently reviewed everything that had happened to me since the examination by Dr. Mines.

I thought about my first visit to the coronary care unit; about my first experience of having an intravenous needle inserted into one of my veins; the weeks of confinement to my hospital bed; of my joy at finally being able to walk around the room; and of my hope that I would soon recover dashed by that initial attack of angina pectoris. I continued to think about the strong attack two days later, which had sent me back to the coronary care unit; of the subsequent daily attacks, which occurred with less and less provocation; and about the ambulance trip to the medical center.

I continued to think about my state of shock when I was told what was actually in store for me; about being prepared for the operation; and about being placed upon that x-ray table in order to undergo the angiocardiographic examination. I thought about the numbing sensation that I felt in my right arm and hand just before I had the stroke; about my heart beating wildly and not pumping the blood to my body as it fibrillated; and about my subsequent journey through the valley of death, which few living men had been able to take. I also thought about the agonizing pains I had endured since that experience and about my inability to swallow or speak. I thought, too, of the endless attacks of angina that were now coming without any provocation.

I could only guess how long I had been lying there in that condition—for weeks, perhaps months. Kept in a drugged, semiconscious state, only interrupted by momentary interludes of conscious wakefulness, I couldn't fully comprehend that I had first been admitted to the intensive care unit less than two short days before. And as I thought about the past and present, I wondered what the future might hold for me —possibly death, more probably the prospect of physical handicap and incapacity.

I lay there considering whether the fight to live was worth all the pain and agony I was enduring. I believed I had actually known what it felt like to die while lying on that x-ray table. I speculated that death might have been the solution to all my afflictions. I reasoned that if I were to close my eyes just then I could take that same trip—but this time to its final destination. No more pain or suffering. No more frustration. Just eternal, peaceful slumber.

I thought about my wife and children, and the insurmountable problems that would plague them if I were gone; of their love; and of their insecurities and fears. My wife would have to lie in an empty bed all alone night after night. And the children—what would become of them, so young to suddenly be left alone? I thought about my daughters creeping into my bed during those rainy nights when the thunder rolled across the heavens into their bedroom. My boys—we were always so close. I was not only their father, but also their friend and mentor. They would have nobody in whom to confide those little problems which only I seemed to understand.

Picturing each one of them pleading with me, calling for me to come home, I decided that life was the challenge—not death. And I knew somehow that I must live, not for myself, but for them. I was then determined that I should live. I so desperately wanted to live.

Although I didn't realize the importance of my decision at the time, my attitude was half the battle in curing me. If I hadn't decided I was going to live, this book would never have been written. But if I was to fulfill my determination to live, I realized that I would have to seek help from other sources.

Granted that I was in a weakened condition from the long period of hospitalization, dieting, sedation and the complete inability to swallow. On the other hand, science had done everything possible to sustain me; oxygen was constantly being supplied to me; some solution in a bottle hanging next to my bed was always being fed to me through the intravenous needle; and the latest drugs and equipment were available for my use. But both sides of the ledger sheet were not balanced.

I did not have the strength to battle for my life in the next round of this important fight and I cast about for another source of strength upon which to draw. And then I knew that my only chance for survival was to summon an ally who knew all about death and life, an ally upon whom I knew I could depend. I prayed to God.

As a Jew, I recited the ancient declaration of faith that all Jews have been reciting since the time of Moses—the declaration of belief in the magnitude and glory of God as the Supreme Being which, through the centuries, gave them the courage to face torture, death and degradation with dignity. *Shema Yisroel, Adonoi Elohanu, Adonoi Echad* (Hear, O Israel, the Lord is Our God, the Lord is One). All through that long night, I kept repeating in my mind this declaration of faith, for I was unable to move my lips to utter the words. Blotting out all other thoughts, I concentrated with passion upon these simple phrases.

Sometime later, still in the early hours of the morning, I awoke from my semiconscious state in the throes of agonizing pain, but still repeating this declaration of my faith in God. Sue was immediately at my bedside, in her hand a hypodermic syringe filled with that merciful Demerol. And as I again started to slip into that twilight sleep, my mind kept repeating over and over again, *Shema Yisroel, Adonoi Elohanu, Adonoi Echad.*

I awoke about 8 A.M. that Thursday morning, September 16, and was startled to find my wife bending over me, the cardiologist and his staff standing at her side. She was smiling and repeating over and over again, "It's a miracle. Lou, it's a miracle."

My mind was still fogged from the last injection of Demerol. I could only blink my eyes and gaze at her. She related how the doctors had just informed her that I had experienced my heart attack during the early morning hours; that ever since the resident doctor had informed them of my severe angina attack the previous night, they had been keeping a close watch by my bedside; that they had instructed the night nurse to keep me completely sedated; and that I was, as yet, unaware of what had happened. Moreover, instead of my having suffered extensive damage to my heart muscle, as was originally feared, the electrocardiograms revealed the area of damage to be comparatively small. And although I would still be in critical condition for the next seventy-two hours, my life no longer hung in the balance. The supposedly fatal heart attack that had been expected to cause extensive damage to a large area of my heart muscle had not occurred.

The cardiologist confirmed her story, adding that I should no longer feel the chest pains of angina because the narrowing artery had now become completely blocked, causing the muscle cells fed in that particular area to become deprived of oxygen and die, so they would no longer cry out for oxygenated blood. He continued that within the next seventy-two hours a scar would start forming over the damaged area, my collateral arteries would begin to grow and eventually take over the feeding of that area of my heart muscle as I convalesced.

I knew that my secret ally had given me the strength and capability to endure the battle for my life.

8 THE AFTERMATH

Although the stroke had left me still speechless, I was over-joyed to learn that I had survived the supposedly fatal heart attack and would soon be able to return to an almost normal life. I wanted desperately to believe in what had occurred in those early morning hours, but I could not at first accept it. What had just been revealed to me by my wife, and confirmed by the doctors, seemed so far-fetched that I could not help but repeat over and over again to myself, "It was a miracle—*a miracle!*"

For the first time since I had arrived back in the intensive care unit, I noticed that I did not feel any of those agonizing pressures and pains building up inside my chest, which had seemed to squeeze the life out of me.

Slowly, by almost imperceptible steps, a feeling of victory and accomplishment pervaded my entire body and every thought. I had won. I was not going to die after all. I would not have to subject myself to any more pain, torture, tests or surgery. In the ecstasy of my thought I bordered on delirium.

After my wife and the doctors had left, I lay on my back, speculating about what had really happened. Then I under-stood that there must be a power in the universe stronger than mortal man. Whether God was some spirit or superior being or just an internal motivating expression of thought, my faith in Him had given me the ultimate strength to overcome death.

The pressures and pains that had kept spreading across my breast were now replaced by a dull throbbing ache immediately over the middle of my chest. I felt as if a baseball had recently ripped through the center of my heart, but the pain was minimal.

Assuming that this mild continuing pain was caused by the damage (infarct) to my heart muscle resulting from the heart attack, I selfishly cherished the ache as if it were my own personal property. It was the symbol of my triumph over death. Consequently, I never told anyone about it.

Throughout the remainder of that day, and during most of the following night, I held my hand over my left breast, gently and slowly massaging it toward the center of my chest. This was a reflex that I was to perform unconsciously almost daily for many months as if to reassure myself that my heart was still functioning smoothly.

When any of the nurses tried to turn me from one side to the other, I balked and would not be moved except to lie on either my right side or back. I refused to lie on my left side or flat on my stomach for fear that my heart would be crushed and stop beating. I didn't discuss this peculiarity with anyone. However, within a matter of several days after the attack, sound reasoning prevailed, and I was able to overcome this block without any help from others.

Although I had experienced the heart attack and had survived, I was not yet past the danger zone in which aberrations in the rate or rhythm of my heartbeat could occur. For seventy-two hours my heartbeat was monitored; oxygen was fed to me; and I was made to feel as comfortable as possible.

In that period of time, as the cardiologist had told me, scar tissue would start to form over the damaged area of the heart muscle, and once dormant coronary blood vessels would awaken to begin the task of replacing the blocked coronary artery (collateral circulation).

I was able to take note, for the first time, of my surroundings. I no longer feared the steps of the doctors and nurses rushing to assist some poor unfortunate patient in that room, or the thumping sound made by the defibrillator as it shocked back to normal another heart that was beating wildly. But I found that I could not control my emotions.

Any news from home, cards from well-wishers, telephone messages from close friends and family, all had to be withheld from me. For almost no apparent reason, tears would well up in my eyes and I would weep. Visitors were limited to my wife and father, and all mail was kept from me.

Convinced that sleep would be most beneficial to the healing processes, I was determined to keep my eyes closed most of the time and try to sleep. I was likewise convinced that I would thus remain more stable emotionally.

I believed that the night nurse, Sue, was my lucky charm and that night I anxiously waited for her to come on duty. She had become associated in my mind with the miracle that had occurred. After all, she was the first person to make me feel comfortable and relaxed when I had returned to the intensive care unit. She was the person who gave me that final injection of Demerol, with which my angina pains had completely disappeared never to return again. And although she denied having anything to do with my recovery, I superstitiously resolved not to have any other nurse wash or shave me, or otherwise tend to my needs.

Within the next two days following the heart attack, my right leg and arm completely recovered their mobility, but I was still unable to swallow. My vocal cords gradually started to respond and intelligible sounds issued from my previously silent throat. For the first time since my stroke, I was encouraged by the hope that I would be able to speak again.

Although I wanted to surprise Sue when she came on duty that night, she had already read my progress chart and came immediately over to my bed to congratulate me. After washing me early the next morning, she encouraged me to practice the alphabet.

Every waking moment I slowly and painfully vocalized the alphabet, letter by letter. My pronunciation was far from clear, but I was greatly pleased to learn that I would be able to communicate vocally instead of in writing. The next night through our concerted efforts I was able to pronounce the words "nurse," "doctor," "please" and "thank you." For me, it was just the beginning of what I thought I could accomplish.

The hours and days that followed were upsetting. Although I tried to communicate with my wife and the hospital staff, nobody could understand what I was saying. And the more difficult it was for anybody to understand me, the more emotionally upset and frustrated I would become. Tears that I was not able to suppress would come to my eyes and roll down my cheeks. Not only was I unable to speak, but I still had to be fed intravenously because I could not swallow. I had not had any food or liquids since coming to the medical center.

One afternoon, forty-eight hours after my heart attack, the patient in the bed next to mine was being served lunch.

Trying not to look at the tray, I had turned my head so that my face was to the wall, but I could not prevent myself from overhearing his conversation with the dietician.

He was complaining because the soup did not contain any salt, and that he would not drink soup without salt. The dietician, trying to coax him into sipping a few spoonfuls of the saltless soup, was offering him a fresh banana as a reward. Unable to contain the rage welling up within me, I suddenly burst into tears. The words that I could not utter reverberated inside my head. I could not understand why a person had to be coaxed into drinking saltless soup, when all that I wanted at that very moment was to quench my parched throat and lips with one solitary drop of water.

Although the fight back to recovery and physical and emotional normality would be quite difficult, I was determined to return to my home and legal practice. I knew that the aftereffects of the stroke combined with the aftereffects of the heart attack would make the task almost insurmountable. But I was not to be daunted. My assets were my determination and the ability to think clearly and rationally.

The first step was the most difficult—to occupy my time so that I would not lapse into a state of depression.

The stroke had not only damaged the speech center of my brain but it had also distorted the vision in my right eye so that I could not read. Radios and televisions were forbidden in the intensive care unit because of the delicate electronic equipment. And I was not able to sit or otherwise get off the bed.

I realized that I would have to concentrate on some subject, other than my ills and complaints, in order to pass those hours when sleep was impossible. It occurred to me that I could plan a book, a book which would be beneficial to mankind.

I would lie on my bed planning such a book, chapter by chapter, sequence by sequence. The research would come at a later time, and so, of course, would the writing. But my waking hours were usefully occupied for many days and weeks.

Most other waking hours were spent in practicing the letters of the alphabet and in improving the verbalization of those few words that I felt I could pronounce. Although I worked hard, my speech improved at a snail's pace. But it was improving, and I was almost able to make myself understood—almost, but not quite. When I grew weary of practicing my speech, I would drift off contentedly into the planning of the book.

On Sunday morning, September 19, three days after I had experienced my heart attack, the oxygen was removed and I knew that I was out of danger. The intern cautioned that removal of the oxygen would cause me to salivate normally again. Until then, my mouth and throat had been dry and I did not have to contend with the problem of swallowing my own saliva. Explaining to me that my throat muscles would gradually come back into use, he told me to swallow the saliva easily and slowly so that I would not strain the dormant throat muscles or choke on my own saliva.

Later that morning, the first few drops of saliva dripped from my salivary glands into my mouth and I swallowed them easily. For the first time since coming to the medical center, I was able to swallow. I waited impatiently to repeat the performance.

During the rest of that day, I lay on my bed in a state of

ecstasy. I now knew that it would be only a matter of time before I would be able to eat and drink again—and perhaps even to talk.

I eagerly waited for Sue to arrive that night. Glowingly she entered with my chart in her hand and informed me of the astounding progress I had made. She agreed to ask the doctor if she could try giving me some water in the morning. The excitement of the day had made me weary, and I knew I would sleep well that night. Before going to sleep, I prayed silently that I would be able to swallow the water if and when it was given to me.

I awoke at 6 A.M. and had Sue wash my hands, face and body and shave my beard. After combing my hair, she used a cotton swab dipped in a special mouthwash to clean my teeth and gums. Sue then changed my bed linens and cranked up the bed to a half-sitting position.

What a difference a few days had made in the state of my physical well-being and mental attitude! I had regained some of my old self-confidence. I still clung to the belief that Sue was my lucky charm and implored her not to desert me.

She hurried over to the doorway and engaged the intern in conversation as he stepped into the room. As they walked slowly to my bedside, I became apprehensive, intense and anxious.

Dear God, I thought to myself, would I at last be able to swallow again? Sue had persuaded the intern to test my throat muscles and I felt myself breathing rapidly.

The intern inserted into my open mouth a long, thin stick with cotton wrapped around one end , and proceeded to dab gently at my throat muscles. At first I was tense and felt nothing. As I relaxed, I could feel the cotton swab gently brushing the muscles way down there inside my throat. He handled the cotton swab so dexterously that I didn't gag. Then he had Sue bring a paper cup half filled with water. She whispered, "Sip this very slowly; do not hurry, no matter how long it will take."

Sipping the water a drop at a time, lest it go down my windpipe (trachea) instead of my food pipe (esophagus), I managed to empty the cup. It had taken a half hour to drink this much water, but I felt as though I had accomplished one of the most difficult trials of my life. I wanted to scream with joy and dance about. Instead I chuckled inwardly and gently squeezed Sue's hand. My lucky charm had not failed me. Now that I was able to swallow, I could be discharged from the intensive care unit that day.

I could not contain my excitement at actually being discharged to a separate room. It would mean that I had passed the seventy-two-hour danger period; it would mean that I would soon be able to sleep undisturbed by the constant *beep-beep-beep-beep-beep* of the monitor; it would mean that I no longer had to be aware of the endless procession of emergency cases; it would mean that the ever-present intravenous needles no longer had to be inserted into my badly bruised and abused veins. I could soon drink liquids, and maybe even eat and talk. I was at last on the road to recovery.

It had been only six days since the ambulance brought me to the medical center. The fight with death and all the pain and suffering I endured were just memories.

I was very weak. I had been in bed for the past thirty-one days, subsisting on various low-calorie diets or nothing at all. I was still depressed and cried almost constantly, but more and more often it was with the sweet tears of joy. I would soon be able to rejoin my loved ones at home and resume an almost normal pattern of life. At four o'clock that afternoon I was discharged from the intensive care unit to a private room in the medical wing of the hospital. I was grateful to find that the room did not contain any oxygen unit or monitoring device. I felt that I had just taken a giant leap to the world of relative safety and comfort.

I was not yet able to cope with the world of reality. My speech had improved to the point where I could make myself intelligible, but I could not talk normally. My right eye was still weak and I could not read for any length of time. I was still emotionally taut. I wanted to hide myself from the outside world and never leave the confines of that hospital room. I was a freak. Having no patience for people who didn't pretend to understand what I was saying, I would ignore them either by turning my face to the wall or by burying my head under the sheet. Many times I asked my wife to leave and never return. I had the television and telephone disconnected, the mail rerouted to my home, and visitors restricted to my wife and my father.

Fifteen minutes after I was settled in the comfortable hospital bed, the head nurse, a stocky, good-natured Irish woman, assured me that I would have the best of care, and in a few days, I would not only be able to eat and drink normally, but also be able to get out of bed. She told me I must drink as much water, apple juice and ginger ale as I could within the next two days. An hour later, she came back into the room with a large trayful of paper cups filled with medication. She handed two of the paper cups to me, one containing water and the other a pill. Although I accepted the pill, I did not have the courage to attempt to place it in

105

my mouth, but she coaxed me into swallowing it. This small pill was the first solid matter to slide down my throat since I had arrived at the medical center. I burst into tears. After I recovered myself, I drained the water from the cup.

It had been a very exciting, but most tiring day for me. Alone in my room, I turned on the radio and heard music, closed my eyes, and went to sleep. For the first time in approximately two weeks I slept soundly and peacefully.

I gazed about the room when I awoke. The reality of the past two weeks' nightmare kept flashing through my mind. I kept thinking about those awful chest pains that had been responsible for my transfer to the medical center. I felt humble and grateful for not having succumbed to the worst.

I also knew that I myself would have to learn to swallow, see clearly and talk. I forced myself to drink a half cup of either apple juice or water every hour. Every time I took two or three sips, my shrunken stomach would be filled to capacity. The next day I forced myself to drink seven cupfuls of apple juice. I knew that soon I would be ready for a normal liquid diet.

The next morning the nurse removed the intravenous needle. That afternoon I was served my first liquid meal of juice, milk, Jell-o, custard and a purée of fruit. I sipped, sucked down and ate my first meal. Finishing the last morsel, I went to sleep.

I was informed that my recovery depended on my getting plenty of rest and not allowing myself to become emotional. I had an idea. I asked my wife to get a book written by William L. Shirer entitled *The Collapse of the Third Republic,* the history of France from the 1870s until the fall of the Republic to the Nazis in 1940. Although my right eye was somewhat strained, I devoured it page by page until I was completely lost in the politics and history of France.

Thus did I overcome my depression, boredom and irritability. I found that the muscles of my right eye were responding to constant reading and were correcting themselves. When I was tired, I drifted off for short naps.

As the days went by, I grew stronger. I found that I could manipulate my mouth and tongue so that I could mash and swallow soft foods. Two weeks later I was able to chew, and was given a regular diet.

That first meal consisted of sliced chicken breast, mashed potatoes, diced carrots and two slices of white bread. Like a baby taking its first steps, I chewed over and over again the bits of chicken and bread for fear that I would choke. And, as the baby learns that it can walk, I discovered that I could chew and swallow.

In the meantime firm scar tissue had formed over the damaged area of my heart muscle. I was in need of much physical rest, but the time had come for me to exercise my body by walking.

As with all hospital patients who have been bed-ridden for any length of time, I could only dangle my feet for the first few days. Then, with assistance from my wife or the nurse, I was permitted to stand on the floor, take one or two steps in the room, and sit in a large chair for short periods of time. Within a few days I could walk about my room and was allowed to go to the bathroom. Before long I was walking in the hospital corridors.

I was able to make myself understood in conversation, but I still had difficulty controlling the right side of my tongue and the right side of my mouth. The fear of not being able to speak fluently made me shut myself up like a hermit. But with the assistance of a speech therapist, I began tongue, lip and mouth exercises. These exercises consisted of licking the outside extremities of the lips with the tip of the tongue; protruding the tongue and then trying to touch my nose and my chin with its tip; and pursing my lips and rotating them in a simulated chewing pattern, clockwise and counterclockwise.

Sitting in the chair or lying on the bed, I would practice these exercises night and day.

The speech therapist was so pleased with my progress that she started me on verbal exercises. I slowly practiced the vowels, then formed and pronounced some of the hard and short letters of the alphabet, such as *g, d, k, t* and *s.* I was especially pleased when I had mastered this phase of the therapy, because I could pronounce words like "good," "kid," "kits," and "dog." I sensed that the time for my discharge had approached, but I feared leaving the haven that the hospital provided. I was still in the grip of emotional depression. My mouth was still distorted and I couldn't pronounce most consonants and vowels distinctly.

On October 8, just forty-nine days after I had been hospitalized, the cardiologist told me I was going to be discharged the next morning.

I hadn't seen any of my children since I left home on that fateful August morning. I wondered how they would react to me. I told my wife the news about my being discharged. We discussed the impact upon the children and decided that my two sons (twelve and fourteen years old) would help bring me home. I asked my wife to bring some toys for my little girls.

Late into the evening, I was restless with excitement and apprehension. With the aid of a sedative I drifted off to sleep.

⑨ GOING HOME

I gazed about the room. This was the morning. I was at last going home. Fifty mornings had come and gone since I entered the coronary care unit. All those mornings, afternoons, days and nights were behind me.

I had trained myself to think ahead a day at a time. There was no sense in worrying about the future. As I sat in bed, following the morning hospital routine for the last time, I tried to imagine what it would be like to see my children after a lapse of almost two months. What could I possibly say to them? Could their young minds grasp the abyss of my experience? My children were only the first step in this transformation back to reality. There would be the neighbors, the relatives, the friends and my business associates.

Would I ever again measure up to being the head of the household, the normal mate, the breadwinner, the provider, the man? As I sat eating breakfast, I realized that the stress and strain of the angina pains and subsequent heart attack had still left me emotionally weak and physically inept.

After breakfast, I put on the clothes that had been brought the evening before, packed my pajamas and turned the chair to the window. The familiar figures of my wife and sons came into view. My pulse started beating and my head started to spin.

My sons had been well coached by my wife. Each of them was smiling. Each took my hand, kissed me and said, "Welcome home." No one asked questions. For the first time I felt at ease.

My wife attended to the discharge papers and release. My sons took my small suitcase and helped me into a waiting wheelchair. We went down in the elevator, through the lobby and out of the hospital. During the ride home I suddenly felt the old familiarity and closeness.

But I was once again overcome with that feeling of uncertainty. It was one thing to be with my sons, but what of my daughters, who were only four and seven? What would they say about the somewhat grotesque appearance of my mouth and my not speaking properly?

So I began to panic again. We turned into our street and made a sharp left into the driveway. I was glad none of the neighbors were there.

The front door was opened by my older daughter. Her face broke into a tremendous smile as she chirped, "Welcome home, Daddy. We all love you and have missed you very much." My younger daughter, Sue, peeped out silently from behind her sister. I was pleasantly surprised to find that the front hall had been decorated with paper streamers, ribbons and signs that read "WELCOME HOME, DADDY." I felt as if I had never left home and that all the love and wanting were still there. My tensions were dissipated.

I gave my daughters the toys. They giggled, bubbled with joy and kissed me. Then the little one got up enough courage to say, "I want you to stay home and don't go to the hospital any more, Daddy." I knew I was home to stay, and I told her just that.

My wife helped me up the stairs to my bedroom. In addition to the large bed, the room also contains a comfortable rocking chair, a television set, radio, a small desk and small wall library. Here I was to remain for the next two weeks, eating off a tray, and receiving no visitors.

Occasionally one of the neighbors would catch a glimpse of me through the window and wave. I would just wave back and disappear into the depths of the room.

Exercise consisted of rocking myself, or pacing about the room several times each day. For amusement I would read a book or the daily newspaper, listen to the radio, watch television, or wade through the cards from friends and relations that had been piling up in a cardboard carton for the past two months.

Sleep came easily those first two weeks. I sponged my body every morning before shaving and hardly had sufficient strength to crawl back into bed. But as the days passed I grew stronger and was able to attend to my needs without tiring. I looked forward to resuming my place as the breadwinner of the family.

When I wanted company, my wife and children would come and talk about all the things that happened to them at home, at school and in the world outside. I was coming out of my shell of seclusion, but I still could not speak about the last two months nor reconcile myself to my physical disabilities. I diligently practiced the tongue, lip, mouth and verbal exercises, and looked forward to my visits to Dr. Mines's office and to the speech therapy clinic.

For the first week at home, I preferred to eat alone. The right side of my tongue, palate and lips were still numbed and I had to concentrate hard on chewing and swallowing. Some-

112

times I took too big a mouthful and gagged. As I learned to control the way in which I chewed and swallowed, I became less self-conscious and would have the family join me at mealtime. My wife had been told to serve low-calorie meals that restricted my intake of eggs, butter, beef and whole milk. I would continue to lose weight and eat less food that was high in cholesterol.

At the end of the first week I felt stronger, both physically and emotionally. I began to eat meals in the kitchen with my wife and children. I laughed to think how easy it was to overcome my fears of rejection.

I was still weak and had to stay in bed twelve to fourteen hours every day. But after school each child would seek me out to talk over the day or ask for help in their homework. My wife took over when she noticed that I was becoming tired and fatigued. I would slip away, leaving the remainder of the problems downstairs for my wife to solve. About two months later, when I became physically stronger, I resumed my role as a husband to my wife.

Fourteen days after my return home I had an office appointment with Dr. Mines. How strange it felt to prepare myself for that office visit. It was the same office where over two months before I made that fortunate call before having a heart attack which could have been fatal. As my wife drove me along the highway, I noticed that the leaves were changing to the yellow, orange and red of late October.

I began to meditate on the changes I had weathered during the past two months, and to ask myself the persistent questions: Would I be able to resume my legal practice? What other occupations would I be able to pursue? Would I continue to be a burden on my wife and children?

Marty told me that I had sustained relatively little damage to my heart muscle; that a firm scar was already formed; and that I should be able to return to a normal life within a reasonably short time.

I was to remain on the same low-calorie, cholesterol-free diet, losing as much weight as I possibly could. He would rather see me ten pounds underweight than even one pound overweight, he said. The course of treatment consisted of diet, regular rest, the avoidance of emotional stress, and moderate physical exercise. I was to continue resting in bed twelve to fourteen hours each day, read, watch television for relaxation, and start a program of gradually increased walking twice a day. Smoking was taboo, and he preferred that I keep alcoholic beverages to a bare minimum.

As we left the office, Dr. Mines handed me two prescriptions, one for a mild sedative called Valium and the other for nitroglycerin. Whenever I felt overwrought, I was to take one of the Valium tablets. If I should ever again experience an anginal pain, I was to slip a nitroglycerin tablet under my tongue and sit down or rest until the tablet had dissolved.

I begged my wife to let me begin the walking exercises immediately. I felt like a child who has just been accepted by one of the school teams. Luckily, I was restrained by my wife. She was acutely aware of the cardinal principle in the convalescence of the heart attack victim, to pace oneself.

Like a benevolent tyrant, she coaxed me into my bed, where I soon fell asleep. In my joy at realizing that I would not be a cripple, I had overlooked the fact that the morning's experience had exhausted me. I slept soundly until supper-time.

The next morning, with the bottle containing the nitro-

114

glycerin tablets in my breast pocket, I gingerly took the initial steps from my house. I felt like a pilot soloing for the first time—unsure of myself, but determined to do what I had set out to accomplish. Slowly and carefully I traversed the thirty feet from the outside door of my home down the driveway to the sidewalk below, the additional fifty feet to my neighbor's driveway, then I turned around and came back again. My wife then helped me to the couch, where I lay for the next hour to regain my strength. I was exhilarated. I repeated the performance that afternoon.

The next day I increased the distance by walking two houses down and back. Each succeeding day I added to that distance by an additional house. I exercised this way twice each day, morning and afternoon, preferably before breakfast and supper. If I exercised following any meal, I was careful to wait for at least two hours. The doctor had explained that the heart pumps extra blood to the digestive system to help digest a meal. If I exercised immediately after eating, my heart would have to pump more blood to my legs and muscles too. Thus I would be putting an extra burden on my heart.

With each succeeding day I was able to walk farther, until I circled the entire block; then two times around the block, three times around, a half mile, one mile, two. Before I was permitted to go back to work, I was walking about two miles every morning and about two miles each afternoon. After each exercise period I would stretch out on the couch or bed for an hour.

I realized that I would probably have angina pains as the distance I walked was increased—and I was not disappointed. The first time was when I had circled half the block.

115

The pains occurred in my throat instead of across my chest, but I recognized angina as I tried to walk one or two paces farther. I leaned against the trunk of a tree, slipped one of the nitroglycerin tablets under my tongue, and in a moment the pains had disappeared. I recognized the attack and knew that I had the antidote.

Dr. Mines had warned me that I might experience angina attacks as I became more active. He had also cautioned me not to panic and to take a nitroglycerin tablet as often as was necessary. As the days and weeks slipped by, the attacks vanished, never to occur again.

The doctor had also cautioned me to avoid walking out of doors when the temperatures were below forty degrees or when there were brisk winds. He explained that the cold air caused a narrowing of the tiniest arteries of the chest, fingers and toes, which would place a strain on my heart muscles. This in turn would bring on attacks of angina. I bought a bicycle exerciser for cold or windy days and inclement weather and used it always before, *never after,* meals.

I developed an insatiable appetite for reading about heart disease (particularly atherosclerosis—the so-called hardening and narrowing of the coronary arteries). My days were very full. I would do my mouth, tongue and lip exercises daily, practice diction and intonation in front of the mirror several times each day, and visit the speech therapy clinic once a month. I walked or exercised on my bicycle exerciser every morning and every afternoon, slept and rested from twelve to fourteen hours each day, and read voraciously the books my wife brought home from the library.

Intervals between visits to the doctor's office were extended from two to three and then to four weeks. I knew that the damage to my heart muscle was continuing to heal rapidly.

The physical effects of the stroke and the heart attack were gradually overcome, but the mental and emotional problems persisted. I was receiving visitors at home and talking to friends and neighbors, but I still could not discuss my illness with anyone other than my intimate family. Nor could I entertain the thought of returning to work. Yet I could not forget the past twenty years spent building a legal practice, and after I was home from the hospital for about two weeks, I called the office at least once a day. My secretary told me that my partners were attending to court cases or were at business closings, and assured me that the office was operating smoothly. Occasionally my partners would tell me the same thing. I accepted these explanations and refused to probe any deeper into any possible problems at the office. I had not yet learned to pace myself throughout the day, nor had I learned not to set deadlines. But after all, I was just another man with a heart and stroke problem that could and would be adjusted to in the course of living.

My wife and I finally took that vacation to the Bahamas for ten full days of sunshine. We wanted to mix with strangers who knew nothing about me or my condition.

During the first few days we remained relatively alone, enjoying each other without the pressures of home. I was almost able to forget my disabilities as we swam, walked and basked on the shores of our warm tropical island.

At dinner one night, we met a couple who were leaving for home the next day. The husband mentioned that he had had a heart attack several years before. At first he had been afraid to face the world; he was too weak physically, too depressed emotionally, and too fearful of being an invalid. Meeting and talking to other people who had suffered heart attacks made him realize that all these fears were a fiction. They were all successful in leading normal lives once again and he was able to identify with them. Each one belonged to the same exclusive club, which he had just joined, a club that demanded the same high initiation fee of all its members—a heart attack. He had learned, as I would also learn, that every member of that club had wrestled with the same problem—that of adjusting to society once again. I myself began to identify with him and started to discuss my own heart attack. It was easy to talk with someone who understood.

The next night a group of lawyers arrived for a one-week convention. At a cocktail party before dinner, I got into a discussion about state law. One of them noticed my slight speech defect and took me to one side. He too had experienced a stroke. I was amazed. He looked normal in every respect. Assuring me that I had only a slight speech impediment and derangement of my right upper lip, which would be corrected with therapy, he made me promise to talk openly about my stroke whenever it was appropriate. Self-consciousness was the stroke victim's worst enemy. By overcoming the fear of being viewed as a freak, he had been able to make a readjustment to society and was once again happy in his legal practice.

During the remaining days of our vacation I talked freely about my stroke and heart attack and my apprehension about the future. As we boarded the airplane for home, I knew I was ready to return to work.

My transition to the normal life of an employable individual was not very easy. Since I would not drive, my wife had to be my chauffeur for those first weeks after my return to the office. I had to adjust myself to the office routine slowly and carefully, first one or two hours a day and finally seven and eight hours. By the time I began putting in a full day and week, I was driving the car myself.

I was most concerned with my position as a key employee and partner returning to an office from which I had been absent for six months. The resentments, connivings and petty jealousies of those who had had to shoulder the burdens had to be accepted. Moreover, I found that I couldn't return as the strong and ebullient person I had been before. I couldn't speak as a dominant member of the firm. Rather, I had to acknowledge my weakness. I swallowed it.

I resolved to change my way of life and methods of working. I could not change my basic concepts, such as being a neat and orderly person. But I found that I did not have to be the hard-driving perfectionist I had almost killed myself being. I would learn to pace myself, steadily and evenly, through the twenty-four hours in each and every day. The world would have to get to know and accept the new me.

Part of pacing myself was learning to recognize when I was beginning to feel fatigued. When that happened, I would stop all activities and lie down on a couch in my inner office. Even when not tired, I would rest perhaps once or twice a day, trying to forget the problems of home and the business.

Trying to avoid deadlines, I was determined to work in the course of my own time. I managed to learn how to walk at a slower pace but with an even gait. Whenever the day's burdens proved to be too much for me, I took several hours off.

119

At last I knew what the doctors meant by my returning to a normal, fruitful life again. I am now a changed person, physically, mentally and emotionally, and I have come to know and respect the individual that I have become. I am more active physically (exercising almost daily by walking, swimming or bicycling) but, having learned how to pace myself, I am more placid and tranquil.

I have lost twenty-five or more pounds. I have almost completely altered my diet into a more normal pattern of eating, and I enjoy wearing clothes that were always too small for me. Above all, I now visit my doctor for a physical examination at least twice each year.

I have often thought about those dark days when I teetered between life and death. I have contemplated what I could have done to prevent that heart attack.

Perhaps my parents could have taken preventive steps during my childhood by providing a properly balanced diet: skimmed milk as a substitute for whole milk, margarine for butter, lean meats instead of fat, and fewer sweets and starches. Perhaps those fatty streaks could have been prevented from forming in my coronary arteries during the first years of life.

During my teens I should have been encouraged to engage in physical exercises such as walking, jogging, running, swimming and bicycling. Daily exercises such as these would have increased the efficiency of my heart muscle and reduced the cholesterol level of my blood.

My teachers and tobacco advertisers could have warned me about cigarette smoking. I now know that smoking is linked to heart disease. I could not have escaped the hereditary factors. My family was prone to coronary disorders and heart attacks. However, being aware of this problem would have made me conscious of my own stressful personality and emotional make-up. I might have striven to be less tense, less of a perfectionist.

If these precautions did not prevent the heart attack, they might have delayed it until a much later time, when the chances of survival would have been vastly improved because my collaterals would have been more developed.

If the heart attack was predestined, I realize now that I required assistance from sources other than my own strength to survive. I know now that I had to rely on values that have been cherished by the human race for so many centuries— the love of a wife and children, and faith in God.